"If you are a wife w
with your spouse, t
be a practical, encouraging breath of fresh air. J. Parker shares practical steps to help higher desire wives work through their sexual desire differences with their spouse and catalyze mutual, positive change. Just as much as the content, though, I appreciate her grace-laced approach to a touchy subject. Let this book encourage and equip you, and give you hope."

Shaunti Feldhahn, social researcher and bestselling author of
For Women Only and *Secrets of Sex and Marriage*

"As a Christian counselor, I wholeheartedly endorse this transformative book by J. Parker. She skillfully addresses a crucial yet seldom-discussed topic, shedding light on the experiences of higher desire wives. Through her wisdom and personal insights, J reveals the underlying issues behind mismatched sex drives and reassures readers that they are valuable, beautiful, and not alone. Most importantly, she offers hope through faith, reminding us that with God, all things are possible."

Kim Kimberling, PhD, CEO, Awesome Marriage

"This is a very needed and welcome book. As a Christian sex therapist, I work with many couples where the wife is the higher desire spouse and there are very few resources for her. I love J's humor in delivering hopeful and helpful information about such a sensitive topic. Thank you, J, for your honest, authentic, and researched approach. I look forward to owning a copy and recommending this to many wives."

Deborah M. Wade, LPC, LMFT, CST,
Christian sex therapist at ACTSolutions

"Finally, a book that speaks right into the heart of every Christian wife who loves sex and wants more of it with the man she married. If that's you, you won't regret digging into this book. Invest in yourself and your marriage with J. Parker's life-changing insights. You're worth it."

Julie Sibert, Christian author and advocate for healthy
sex in marriage, IntimacyInMarriage.com

"We live in a sex-saturated culture where couples are having far less sex. This pattern is having significant consequences on the health of the connection between husbands and wives. In *The Higher Desire Wife*, J. Parker speaks to an often overlooked aspect of this sexual divide. With practical advice and biblical encouragement, J helps wives know they are not alone. This book will not only encourage you but also point you in a direction toward better intimacy."

Kevin A. Thompson, author of *Friends, Partners & Lovers*

"I hear from many wives who desire more sex and wonder why their husband is not engaging more sexually. J. Parker's encouraging words help such a wife understand what issues may be underlying the sexual disconnect in her marriage, take ownership for what she *can* do, and engage in constructive conversations and actions to maximize the intimacy she is longing for while caring for both her heart and her marriage. Practical and uplifting."

Carol Tanksley, MD, DMin, author of *Sexpectations: Reframing Your Good and Not-So-Good Stories about God, Love, and Relationships*

"J. Parker has written a cutting-edge primer in the field of healthy sexuality. There are not enough resources for the wife who has a high desire to be sexual with her husband! Thank you, J, for providing this thorough look at all aspects of a marriage with a higher desire wife. You provide hope and healing to a neglected population."

Bonny Logsdon Burns, APSATS-CPC, ADOH, ACC, restoration coach, author, and speaker, StrongWives.com

"J. Parker finally addresses the one nagging question we hear all the time from higher drive women: 'What's wrong with me?' With the patience and understanding of a woman who's been there, her clear answers are the sighs of relief that women around the world need to hear."

Brad and Kate Aldrich, Aldrich Ministries Coaching Network

The Higher Desire Wife

The
Higher Desire
Wife

UNDERSTANDING AND HELP FOR CHRISTIAN WOMEN
NAVIGATING MISMATCHED SEX DRIVES

J. PARKER

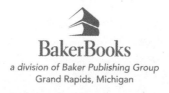

BakerBooks

a division of Baker Publishing Group
Grand Rapids, Michigan

© 2025 by Julie Parker

Published by Baker Books
a division of Baker Publishing Group
Grand Rapids, Michigan
BakerBooks.com

Printed in the United States of America

Library of Congress Cataloging-in-Publication Data
Names: Parker, J., 1967– author.
Title: The higher desire wife : understanding and help for Christian women navigating mismatched sex drives / J. Parker.
Description: Grand Rapids, Michigan : Baker Books, a division of Baker Publishing Group, [2025] | Includes bibliographical references.
Identifiers: LCCN 2024024992 | ISBN 9781540904416 (paper) | ISBN 9781540904744 (casebound) | ISBN 9781493449118 (ebook)
Subjects: LCSH: Man-woman relationships—Religious aspects—Christianity. | Women—Religious aspects—Christianity. | Sex role—Religious aspects—Christianity.
Classification: LCC BT705.8 .P34 2025 | DDC 248.8/435—dc23/eng/20241105
LC record available at https://lccn.loc.gov/2024024992

Some names and details have been changed to protect the privacy of the individuals involved.

Cover design by Rebecca Lown Design
Illustration by Thea McRae

The author is represented by the literary agency of Credo Communications, LLC.

Baker Publishing Group publications use paper produced from sustainable forestry practices and postconsumer waste whenever possible.

25 26 27 28 29 30 31   7 6 5 4 3 2 1

To the women who've been in my higher desire wife community. You make me glad that I went without sex when I really wanted it so that I could understand the plight and launch our cool club. I think . . .

On further reflection, never mind. I'd rather have y'all *and* more sex with my husband.

Still, you're the best. Thanks for sharing your hearts with me.

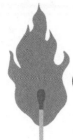

Contents

Foreword

This book is about to become one of your favorite resources as you navigate this journey of being a higher desire wife. I'm sure of it.

I had the pleasure of meeting J through the wonderful world of social media. And through that same platform, we formed a friendship and became colleagues led by our mutual hope and desire to bring healing to people—especially women—who struggle in their marital intimacy. I've had the honor of having several personal conversations (not always about sex) with J, and time and time again she has proven her giftedness, her heart, and her calling around Christ-focused sexual wholeness. She has also shown that well in this book.

Reading this book is like having coffee (or hot tea if you're not a coffee lover) with a more experienced and wiser sister, an understanding therapist, a mature Christian, and that one cousin who gives you the actual deets of how the body works. A strange combination, perhaps, but one you'll enjoy even though you didn't know it was the very thing you were looking for.

J does a beautiful job of making you pause to consider all the factors that could potentially play a role in the desire discrepancy between you and your hubby, sometimes with research and interesting facts, and other times with thought-provoking comments and statements. Considering those statements, this book can be a bit difficult to read. But let's be real. The whole situation of being a higher desire wife is challenging, so thinking about it and talking about it will be challenging as well.

The beauty in this book is that while J will challenge you to make some changes in your behavior and thoughts, she does it with such grace, kindness, personal stories (her own and others'), and humor that it's a pretty satisfactory journey.

Finally! A book that helps the higher desire wife not feel broken, shamed, or alone. Instead, J walks alongside you, reminding you that not only are you not broken, shamed, or alone, but you can work toward a happier marriage and find peace with your higher sex drive.

As a certified Christian sex therapist, I was impressed to see that J did not simply offer some encouragement or build her ideas around her own life or her work with others. While she shares all that knowledge, she also did her research to make sure that she offers solid, helpful advice. She gives examples of when a wife or couple might want to seek the help of a licensed counselor, and she offers a balanced mix of research and a theological view of what your unmet desires mean for you, as well as how to handle these drives in ways that honor the God who gave them to you.

I really enjoyed reading J's book and am so happy for you, my sister in Christ, that you've also found this book. May you be blessed, and may the Lord give you strength, peace, grace, and wisdom as you read J's words and practice the concepts she teaches you.

Your fellow sojourner,

Dr. Jessica McCleese
Licensed clinical psychologist and
certified Christian sex therapist

Being a Higher Desire Wife

What's an acceptable level of sexual desire for a wife? Or any woman? For a long time, I couldn't answer that question well. And for me, the confusion began in my teens. Let me set the scene.

I'm sixteen years old. It's a Wednesday night. I sit in an upstairs classroom in my church with two Bible class teachers. These middle-aged women are here to share their wisdom with teenage girls beginning to explore romantic relationships: "Boys want sex. When you're on a date and they try something, you have to be the one to stop things from going too far."

My stomach tightens; my mind churns.

Why is everything up to me? What am I—a chastity traffic cop? So he gets to shift into gear with his sex drive while I have to control my urges and stop him too? What if I have a strong sex drive?

Wait—does me having as strong a sex drive as the guy make me a freak show? Or worse . . . a slut?

What They Didn't Understand

My teachers didn't know the effect their words would have on sixteen-year-old me, or on any other girl in the class who felt as I did. Presumably, these women had lower libidos than their husbands and believed that encouragement to remain pure was sufficient to keep us on the right path. Moreover, these well-meaning women parroted a common thread that has run through churches and secular circles for many years: the belief that women simply aren't as sexually driven as men.

The vast majority of marriage resources, TV and media, and common conversations iterate this same perspective. Often the message goes like this: men want sex, women want romance.

For Christians following the no-sex-before-marriage plan, this means that women can get what they want before and after the "I dos," while men must wait until the knot is tied to get their goody. But then—watch out! Because the beast has been unleashed and needs to be fed.

What happens for the wife who gets married and discovers that was a big fat lie? The Christian wife with a strong sex drive who looks forward to sex, only to find her husband less interested than her? Or that wife who didn't have the stronger sex drive when she married but years later finds herself far more eager to make love?

Instead of a beast, her husband seems sexually tamer than a caged hamster.

Why Not Flip the Advice?

"Just flip it!" some say. "If you want sex more than he does, read the usual advice and substitute 'wife' where it says 'husband,' and vice versa." Then her voracious desire is the beast unleashed, right?

But many wives with high sexual interest and a lack of reciprocity don't feel like sexy beasts but rather beasts of burden. Their strong libido can seem like a weighty load, and they worry that they are undesirable, feel guilt for being "too much," or harbor resentment that they were dealt this unexpected and unwanted hand. Such unique feelings are not well addressed, or even acknowledged, in many marriage resources.

Moreover, a higher desire wife is still a woman. W-O-M-A-N. Her physiology, emotion, and perspective reflect her femaleness, so a lot of the advice given to higher desire husbands simply doesn't fit wives. For instance, a higher desire woman can be mentally raring to go, while her body requires more lead-up and foreplay than a higher desire man's.

And her husband is still a man, with his reasons for not sexually engaging overlapping with those of lower desire wives but having distinct features and consequences. From his different hormones to cultural expectations and more, a lower desire husband's experience doesn't correspond perfectly with a less interested woman's.

You can't simply flip the advice like a flapjack. Higher desire wives face a unique situation that deserves its own special treatment. That special treatment is what I've long wanted to give.

Why I Wrote This Book

In late 2010, I started a blog called *Hot, Holy & Humorous* in which I wrote primarily to wives, helping them understand and embrace God's design for sex in marriage. Just over a year into my ministry, I wrote my first post about higher desire wives (HDWs). It hit home with many women, and I began hearing from them—all stories that I had great compassion for.

I continued to write posts for HDWs and launched a Facebook group for these women that attracted over seven hundred members before I had to shut it down due to security issues. After that, I founded a subscription community for HDWs to find information, advice, and encouragement. I also spoke about higher desire wives on my popular podcast, *Sex Chat for Christian Wives*, cohosted by Bonny Burns, Chris Taylor, and until recently Gaye Christmus. And I appeared on others' podcasts on the topic, hoping to bring awareness and insights to couples with a sexual desire discrepancy that leans toward the wife wanting more sex.

Still, I wanted to do even more. I wanted to create a resource that higher desire wives could turn to—that spoke to their unique experience and provided a framework for why and what next. I felt God's pulling on me to write a book.

Even though I'd spent a lot of time and effort learning about HDWs, I wanted to cover the subject as thoroughly as possible. So I spent hours upon hours researching the reasons for desire differences, practical ways to address obstacles, and especially the Bible's word on the matter. And I scheduled interviews with several HDWs (mostly tapped from my higher desire wife community), whose stories are woven into the book where applicable.

How This Book Will Help

The primary goals of this book are:

- to show you that you're not alone
- to help you identify the underlying reasons for the desire gap between you and your husband
- to provide information, insight, and practical steps to address each of those reasons
- to encourage Christian virtues such as love, kindness, and patience throughout this process
- to deepen your understanding of God's design for sex, both broadly and for your specific marriage

We'll begin in part 1 with understanding the issue, then move on in part 2 to reasons why your husband may have a lower drive. In part 3, we'll tackle why your drive is higher, and in part 4, I'll provide practical tips for addressing the desire discrepancy. In part 5, I want to leave you with genuine hope for satisfying sexual intimacy.

Can you resolve the gap and enjoy a holy, healthy, and happy sex life with your husband? Yes! There are no guarantees—oh, how I wish there were!—but doing nothing gets you nowhere, while doing something is far more likely to yield results you want.

Your willingness to diagnose the issues, to take action when possible, and to pursue deeper intimacy with your husband is key to making progress.

What God Knows

> You have searched me, LORD,
> and you know me. (Ps. 139:1)

If only I'd believed that Scripture as I sat in my dating-wisdom class at the tender age of sixteen. I ached to feel that someone knew me, understood me, loved me for who I was.

That's also what my twenty-six-year-old self, my thirty-six-year-old self, and my forty-six-year-old self wanted to believe—that God knew the sexually driven woman I was and valued me.

It's what many wives reading right now desperately desire. You haven't felt known. Too often, your situation has been ignored, belittled, or given a passing nod.

Not here, my dear, lovely friend. God knows.

I know who you are too. Because, *psst*, I am one of you—a higher desire wife. And not just one of you; I'm running for captain of the club. I've been everything in my marriage—equally matched, lower desire for a few years after children came, and higher desire in later years—but my marriage has reflected the higher desire wife / lower desire husband dynamic for over a decade now. I've struggled, but I've learned a lot through my Christian sex ministry, delved deep into a wide array of resources, conversed with wives like you and me, and come to a lovely place in my own marriage in which I don't experience sex as often as I could engage but enjoy a satisfying amount and quality.

You're not alone. There are answers. You can make things better.

UNDERSTANDING THE ISSUE

Before we get into the particulars of your marriage's sexual mismatch and how to address them, let's talk about the issue itself. How prevalent are higher desire wives, what are we talking about when we discuss sexual desire and the gap between husband and wife, and what's all this got to do with God anyway?

1. How Many of Us Are There?

Because the belief that husbands have higher sex drives and wives have lower ones is so prevalent in both Christian and secular culture, many a wife with the opposite experience has felt alone. She's the odd woman out in conversations with other wives, the isolated wife at marriage conferences that cover sexuality, the lonely lover at home wondering who else could possibly understand what she's going through.

Too often, she feels like the awkward kid standing against the wall at the junior high dance, wondering if the event was really meant for her too. Or maybe she misread the invitation.

The older a wife is, the more likely this is true.

Recently, more Christians have addressed the topic of sex in marriage, and within this greater pool of resources, some have acknowledged or somewhat addressed the scenario of a higher desire wife and lower desire husband (LDH). Many younger wives have read or heard about marriages in which he's less interested than her, but a woman who married decades ago likely had few, if any, resources to help her navigate the situation. She bore her secret alone, not knowing where to turn.

The Beauty of Community

Many HDWs experience sweet relief when they discover that they are not alone but exist in a community of women who get it. Here's

21

a sampling of what higher desire wives in my Facebook group shared about finding community:

- "Most Christian books I read on the subject early in our marriage said that husbands want it, wives don't, and you must keep your hubby interested so he doesn't stray. Nowhere did I read the opposite can be true, and what to do about it. It's so *refreshing* to know there are other HD wives who get it."
- "It's weird to long for my husband to desire and pursue me and go around wondering what the heck is wrong with me (or my husband). . . . Knowing other women experience this makes me feel a lot *less alone.*"
- "I cried myself to sleep many nights praying the Lord would take away my desires. Of course due to stereotypes I felt like I must be the only one going through this. I was *encouraged* and *relieved* when I realized other marriages have similar challenges."

You're not the only wife not constantly pursued by her husband. Others have struggled as you have, and some wives have figured out this challenge and can offer ideas and support. You may not have wanted to join the club, but we're all here and you're more than welcome. Wipe your shoes on the mat and come on in.

What Percentage of Wives Are Higher Desire?

As the topic of higher desire wives has begun to be discussed more, various percentages have been kicked around. Sometimes the number is as low as 10%, sometimes as high as 50%, but most often *experts say 15–30% of marriages have a higher drive wife.* Based on spouses I'd heard from, that number sounded about right, but was it? After all, other statistics batted around a lot don't turn out to be true. For instance, the much-touted 50% divorce rate

22

was based on modeling that didn't manifest in real life.[1] Keeping examples like this one in mind, I put on my hunting cap and went searching for the truth.

In 2020, the *Journal of Sexual Medicine* published a study of 2,400 Canadians, ages 40–59, in which the most common sexual problem was low desire, with 40% of women and 30% of men reporting this issue.[2] That statistic aligns with the upper end of the 15–30% estimate and could indicate the estimate was a little low. However, the researchers had asked whether the problem of low drive had occurred anytime during the previous six months, so that percentage captured both perpetually low drive husbands and the equally matched or higher drive husband who has an off day or week.

One 1995 study reviewed the cases of 588 clients seen for hypoactive sexual desire disorder—that is, lack of interest in sex.[3] Among this sample, 19% of participants were male. This sample, of course, involved those who went looking for help, and it's possible that fewer couples with a lower drive husband seek help than those with a lower drive wife.

A 2018 study looked specifically at couples transitioning into parenthood and found that among the 255 couples surveyed, 5% were equally matched, 70% had a higher desire male, and 25% had a higher desire female.[4] How hormonal and life changes impact each gender's desire for sexuality poses an interesting question, but the breakdown seems consistent with other findings.

Perhaps the most comprehensive perspective comes from the British National Survey of Sexual Attitudes and Lifestyles (NAT-SAL), which is carried out every ten years. The most recent published results (2010–12) included 4,839 men and 6,669 women, ages 16–74 years.[5] Among this large sample, 34.2% of women and 15% of men reported a lack of interest in sex for three or more months in the past year. Yet this study polled individuals with one or more sex partners in the prior year, rather than people in marriages or long-term relationships.

One survey repeatedly cited by some, suggesting that women have as high or higher a drive than men, deserved attention. Noting an increase in lingerie and sex toy searches, a private British company commissioned a study of 2,383 Britons in long-term relationships and reported that 57% of women and 41% of men wanted more sex with their partner.[6] However, the original study is not readily available, its sampling cannot be verified, and its findings are an outlier. While it might be tempting for HDWs to claim, "Hey, we're actually a majority!" I don't believe that's true.

In the first draft of this book, I wished for a study of about 5,000 people, equally divided among male and female, married for three-plus years, and reporting on overall sexual interest in their marriage. I lamented that I didn't have a rich, distant relative to leave me a truckload of money to finance that study.

And then came research by certified sex therapist Dr. Michael Sytsma and social researcher Shaunti Feldhahn, with 5,300 people, mostly married, reporting on overall sexual interest in their relationship. (Thanks for that, y'all!) Their study revealed that 21% of couples were equally matched, 54% had a higher desire husband, and 24% had a higher desire wife.[7]

From this data, we can draw some reasonable conclusions. If we toss out the suspect outlier study, the percentages of men with low sexual interest were 15%, 19%, 24%, 25%, and 30%. Apparently, that's where we get this claim: *experts say 15–30% of marriages have a higher drive wife.*

Having studied this issue extensively, conversed with marriage therapists and ministers, and heard from many husbands and wives, I feel confident that the number is at least 15% of couples, though I think it's likely 20–25%.[8]

Real-Life Implications

In 2022, there were an estimated 61.44 million opposite-sex married couples in the United States.[9] Fifteen percent would be 9.22

million couples with higher drive wives. The slightly higher estimate of 20% would be 12.29 million couples with higher desire wives, and 25% would be 15.36 million couples.

In other words, a lot.

But let's take this down to a more personal level. The next time you sit in church, look around at the married couples and imagine one in five has a higher drive wife. It's true also at your workplace, your cooking class, your children's PTA meeting, your nail salon, or wherever else you go: one in five wives there has experienced something like what you have. They get it.

So do I.

Hopefully, you now recognize you're not an oddball, not uniquely challenged, and certainly not alone. We're in this together, so let's start our journey of figuring out what to do with the mismatch of sex drives in your marriage.

2. Sex Is a Two-Player Sport

You're higher drive and he's lower drive. But what does that mean? After all, "higher drive" and "lower drive" are relative terms.

Just like "faster" and "slower" depend on who you're running with while being chased by an angry rhinoceros, "higher" and "lower" depend on who you're comparing with and when. A woman with a higher drive than her husband might have the lower drive if she was married to a different man or in a different season of marriage.

Let's establish, therefore, what sex drive is, when the mismatch between spouses becomes a problem—perhaps not as much as running from a charging rhino, but still—and the goal of closing the gap.

Defining Desire

Several phrases are used to refer to wanting sex: sex drive, libido, sexual interest, sexual desire. While these terms technically describe the same thing, they convey different nuances.

"Sex drive" seems to most like an intense desire to make love before arousal occurs.

"Libido" tends to be seen as the physiological side of sexual desire—how your body clues you into sexual desire and awakens to the idea of lovemaking.

"Sexual interest" more often describes not an independent desire to make love but a willingness to engage—that is, interest in lovemaking whether it comes before or after arousal.

"Sexual desire" is straightforward in meaning, easily understood as wanting sex. Where that longing comes from depends on the individual and the marriage.

You may prefer one term over another, but all will be used in this book. Overall, we'll use these terms in ways that acknowledge that, regardless of where desire originates—from a physical, mental, or emotional place—we're focused on one primary issue: you want sex more than your husband does.

Defining "More"

Most often, "more" means frequency, but it can also refer to the intensity of desire or the longing to expand your sexual repertoire. For example, you may be having sex as often as you'd like, but you're doing most or all of the initiating or he doesn't seem to enjoy it as much as you do. You long to be sexually desired at the same level that you desire your husband.

Or you may be tired of the same old routine: kiss like that, touch right here, use that one sexual position, A-B-C, X-Y-Z. You know that sweet sensations are available for your pleasure and his, if only you two could get out of that rut. But he's not interested in changing his approach.

Whatever it means to you to want sex more—frequency, intensity, or receptivity to new experiences—if your longing is greater than his, you qualify as a higher desire wife.

The Width of the Gap

While higher desire wives all agree with the statement "I want sex more than he does," some want it slightly more than their husband, others experience a bigger gap, and some have a chasm so large they haven't had sex in years.

How much work you have to do depends in part on where you start. If the gap is narrow, you may find the answers quickly and move into a better place with some intentionality. If the gap is wide, you may have more than one issue to address, need to whittle away at the problems, or even need to seek professional help.

Most HDWs reading this book will fall somewhere in between—needing some insight, personal effort to make changes, and perseverance to keep improving.

Also, the width of the gap can and will likely change. A wife's desire may be higher or lower depending on the season of marriage, but so may a husband's desire.

Regardless of where you begin, you can make progress. This book will help you figure out how to move forward.

Your Husband's Part

Another important factor in how quick, complete, and lasting your progress will be is your husband's willingness to take part. Most lower interest spouses have little to no idea what sex means to you—that is, how much that particular kind of intimacy impacts you feeling loved and secure in the marriage.

Your husband is likely oblivious rather than malicious. Because his urges are not as strong as yours, he struggles to understand what it feels like for you. For men in particular, it can be difficult to confront a woman's stronger desire, since that can make him feel like he doesn't measure up (a topic we'll cover more in a later chapter).

As we go, we'll talk about how to get him on board as much as possible. The more a wife can involve her husband, the easier it will be to align their sexual satisfaction. But since sex is a two-player sport, he has a choice in this too, and you want to persuade rather than drag him to the bedroom.

At least, I hope you do. Though you may have considered dragging him a time or two.

What God Desires

If sex is a two-player sport, it's one with an amazing coach. Not only is God our perfect coach for life, including our sex lives, he invented the game! He wants it to be played and played well.

Throughout this book, we'll look at what God says in the Bible about sexual intimacy in marriage. He says that it's for reproduction, enjoyment, and marital intimacy for both husband and wife. You can delve much deeper into God's many purposes and desires for sex with my devotional book, *Biblical Intimacy: A Wife's Devotional Journey to Better Sex in Marriage*.

We'll explore God's teachings and how his commands can guide our steps as we progress toward better unity regarding sex in our marriage. For now, let me suggest that the most important verse in the whole Bible about sex isn't in 1 Corinthians 7 (a well-known chapter on marriage), Proverbs 5–6 (a passage advising faithfulness to one's spouse), or even Song of Songs (a whole book dedicated to marital passion). Rather, it's a verse in Philippians about Christ's humility: "Let each of you look not only to his own interests, but also to the interests of others" (2:4 ESV).

It's fine to look to your own interests, such as your sexual desire for your spouse, but you should also attend to the interests of others, including your husband with his lower drive.

And speaking of your husband—that hottie you're hungry for—let's start with why he doesn't want sex as much as you do.

PART 2

WHY IS HIS DRIVE LOWER?

Most higher desire wives start with wanting to know why their husband isn't interested in sex. Is it her? Is it him?

While this part is the largest one of the book, please don't let the number of pages needed to cover this question make you think *he* is the whole problem that needs to be fixed (more on that in the next chapter). Rather, I've included as many reasons as possible, as well as ways to work through those issues. Your husband won't fit all or most of them, but more than one factor often contributes to a husband's lack of sexual interest.

So let's go through the options and discover what might be going on with your beloved.

3. Is Something Wrong?

Anna has smooth skin, bright eyes, a sweet smile, and a trim, curved figure. Raised in a culture that implied men couldn't control themselves sexually, that they were "almost like animals," she was shocked to discover that her husband's sexual interest was significantly less than hers. Not that she wanted an out-of-control animal, but having a man who didn't want sex much threw her for a loop.

Two and a half years later, she described to me her ongoing breakdowns and the self-talk she struggles with that includes statements like "You're ugly" and "You're so pitiful." She looks for distractions and prays for God to take away her sex drive.

But underlying her surprise, her frustration, and her emotional pain is the question she keeps trying to answer: why? Why doesn't her husband desire more sex with his wife?

Paging Dr. House

When the wife has less drive than her husband, society looks on that as typical, expected, something to work on but not necessarily a defect. Yet when it's the husband who has less drive—call the paramedics! Summon Sherlock Holmes! Pray for divine intervention! Bring in Dr. House!

Yes, higher desire wives often wish they had their own Gregory House, MD—the character played by Hugh Laurie in the popular

TV series *House*. Dr. House oversees a team of diagnosticians and regularly demonstrates his incomparable prowess in making the right diagnosis to inform treatment.

If only a higher desire wife could take her list of symptoms to a sex drive diagnostician who could provide the exact reason why her husband desires sex less. Once an accurate diagnosis was delivered, treatment would become clear. And soon the "patient" and his beloved would be celebrating their second-chance revival—by getting busy regularly and happily.

Dr. House is not included within these pages. And when we talk about diagnosing, we're simply trying to figure out why there's a gap between how much a wife and her husband desire sex. We're diagnosing a problem, not a person.

Yet, with the same attention to detail, we'll delve into the myriad causes for a husband's reluctant or absent sexual interest. There could be a sole reason that can be addressed with relative ease, or there could be many that require a multipronged approach. Read each chapter carefully to determine whether and how your story fits.

But remember, we are not our husband's sex doctor and he is not our patient! We want to inform ourselves as best we can about what's going on, but not so we can "fix" him. Rather, we want to partner with our spouse to resolve the sexual desire gap.

Not His Doctor, Not His Coach

Not only are we not our husband's doctor, we're also not his life coach. As you go through these chapters on why your husband's libido isn't firing at your level or above, please don't use them to launch "here's what we need to do" advice for him. Instead, take it all in, mull it over, and pray about it.

If you come upon something likely contributing to your sex drive mismatch, you may feel a sense of urgency to share with him the answers you've discovered and get things moving in a different direction. I get it. Really, I do. I love sharing discoveries with my husband, especially when I believe it could improve our marriage.

But hold your fire for a bit longer and go through parts 3 and 4, "Why Is Your Drive Higher?" and "Now What?" Particularly in the latter, I give invaluable tips on how to communicate effectively with your husband and change the dynamics in your marriage.

Ditch the idea of being his doctor or his life coach. Instead, consider yourself the scout—going ahead, checking things out, and returning to share what you've learned. In the same way that Joshua and Caleb believed that God would give them victory, I'm confident you can make great progress too.

Let's start scouting.

Physical Health

When wives or husbands explain sexual problems and ask for my advice, often the first recommendation I give is for the struggling spouse to see a healthcare provider—a physician, nurse practitioner, or medical specialist. It's important to address or rule out physiological issues.

Even when nonphysical issues need to be addressed—and often they do—it's best to take care of the physical ones up front. Then the spouse or couple can face the other problems with greater energy and wellness.

To that end, let's go through what health issues might impact a husband's sexual interest. And yeah, the list is long.

4. Low Testosterone

One of the most common conversations reported to me by HDWs goes like this:

> Wife: My husband isn't as interested in sex as I am.
> Friend: You should get his testosterone checked. I bet he has Low T.

Yep, that's it—the whole conversation. Low male libido? Get that man some testosterone!

It's not just male supplement ads that make this case. Many men and women believe a husband's comparatively lower sexual desire must be linked to low levels of this male sex hormone.

How often is low testosterone the actual culprit? Not nearly as often as people think. However, checking testosterone levels is one of the first suggestions I give. Why? Because if it is Low T, that physiological issue is easy to resolve, so why go through all the other options?

Why Testosterone Matters

Testosterone is a sex hormone present in both males and females; however, its prevalence is about ten times greater in men.[1] Testosterone plays a role in bone mass, muscle mass and strength, how efficiently fat is burned, sperm production, and, yes, sex drive. It's also implicated in hair growth when a man is younger but balding when he's older.[2] (Go figure.)

As seen by nature's balancing act, it's not just low testosterone that can cause a man problems, but high testosterone as well. Both low and high testosterone can result in low sperm counts, smaller testicles, and impotence. Since no one wants that, we're aiming to keep your gent right there in the sweet spot.

Moreover, not only is the right level of testosterone good for your husband's libido and sexual performance, it's also good for his health. Sweet-spot T helps keep his heart, prostate, bones, muscles, blood pressure, and mood all in good working order.

What's Normal?

A doctor cannot diagnose a man with low or high testosterone without knowing what's standard, or "normal," for him. One would think that answer is straightforward: measure the T, compare it to a chart, and see whether the test shows low, high, or average. But while there are charts used for such a diagnosis, the right amount of testosterone for a man varies depending on many factors.

Still, let's start with the chart. Mount Sinai's School of Medicine suggests the range for normal testosterone in men is 300–1,000 nanograms per deciliter.[3] Labcorp, one of the largest clinical laboratories in the US, breaks down normal male ranges further by age and uses picograms per milliliter (pg/mL):[4]

Age	Range (pg/mL)
0–19	Not established
20–29	9.3–26.5
30–39	8.7–25.1
40–49	6.8–21.5
50–59	7.2–24.0
>59	6.6–18.1

If your husband gets tested for testosterone, his level will be measured against a chart like this one. However, testosterone levels fluctuate across the year and within a day. That is, testosterone can increase or decrease according to seasons and is highest in the morning and lowest in the evening. For that reason, experts recommend a man get tested more than once to confirm levels and have his blood drawn around the same time of day each time. If these recommendations are not followed, you may not get an accurate result.

But even an accurate number may not tell you everything you need to know because a perfectly fine level for one man might be problematic for another. As biochemist Daniel Kelly explains,

> Testosterone takes action when it joins onto its receptor in any particular cell in our body. But how well it does this . . . differs from person to person, which is influenced by genetics. So what might be considered a low level for one person may actually be OK if they have a more sensitive receptor capable of carrying out testosterone's actions at lower concentrations.[5]

If your husband is way outside the normal range, that may indicate his testosterone level is at least a contributor, and addressing that glitch could ramp up his sexual interest. But discovering how much testosterone is right for your husband within the wide range of normal may be a more delicate dance.

So how can you know if his lower sexual desire is a function of Low T? Consider other symptoms. In addition to lowered sex drive, a man with Low T may experience fatigue, irritability, difficulty concentrating, weight gain, or erectile dysfunction. While these can be indicative of other conditions or personal stress, paired with a Low T blood test, a doctor will likely consider or order treatment.

As for High T, that's a less likely cause of libido problems—though it could cause sexual dysfunction, which in turn dampens interest. Symptoms of High T include increased appetite, mood swings, headaches, and uncharacteristic aggression, but once again, proper diagnosis and treatment should involve a health-care professional. Typically, hyperandrogenism, the fancy word for High T, results from certain medications, testosterone supplements, tumors, or pituitary gland diseases—meaning that treatment involves treating the underlying cause.[6]

How to Treat Low T

Let's say your husband believes his testosterone could be low. He may be tempted to skip the medical approach and go for a testosterone supplement. Believe me, there are a gazillion stores that would love to sell your hubby a product that promises to boost his T to TNT levels.

However, not only are such products unlikely to help, but they could also cause other health problems, such as sleep apnea, prostate growth, increased risk of blood clotting, and low sperm production.[7] As noted before, you want to make sure your husband gets the right amount of testosterone—not too much, not too little, but just right. So involve a medical professional to get a proper diagnosis and treatment.

Let's say your husband visits a doctor, has his levels checked, and discovers his testosterone measures on the too-low-to-crow side. What's the next step? Medical professionals address the issue of Low T through testosterone therapy. This includes several options: injections into the bloodstream, gels or solutions absorbed through the skin, tablets applied to the gums that then get into the bloodstream, pellets implanted under the skin, and even a nasal gel pumped into one's nostrils. Each treatment has pros and cons and should be carefully monitored by a healthcare provider to make sure it's working and to avoid side effects.[8]

One last thing: What kind of a doctor should your husband see? A primary care or internal medicine physician can order blood tests and address concerns, but the specialty that testosterone levels fall within is endocrinology.

5. His Weight

When I began researching causes of low sex drive among men, I was taken aback by how often unhealthy weight appeared in my searches. I wondered, *Why isn't this being talked about more?* But of course it isn't. No man wants to be told that, on top of not being up to snuff in the sexual interest area, he needs to go on a diet.

Even as I begin this chapter, I'm nervous to tackle this topic for fear of coming across as fat shaming or setting unrealistic expectations for people who struggle with weight gain. Both men and women are regularly targeted with messaging about the problems of excess weight, and some messages are delivered in a less-than-helpful spirit. Please hear my heart before we jump in here: this is not about anyone who is overweight but healthy! And lots of plus-sized couples have satisfying sexual intimacy.

But not everyone does. Some husbands are not experiencing their best sex life because their weight has reached an unhealthy point for their specific body to engage.

The Risks of Obesity

Urologist Jamin Brahmbhatt put it simply: "It is commonly known that obese men have lower levels of testosterone."[1] As covered in the last chapter, testosterone is a key hormone for sparking sex drive.

Even if your husband doesn't qualify as obese, an increasing waist-line, specifically when paired with poor calorie choices, could lead to lower testosterone in the future. Moreover, since we don't know exactly the right amount of testosterone for any particular man, obesity could lower a hubby's T just enough to pour water on that spark.

But even if testosterone is flooding his system, having sex requires energy, endurance, and blood flow—three requirements negatively impacted by obesity. It's just plain physics that it takes more effort to move a larger object, so if a man is sporting more pounds than his muscles can easily lift, then sex can sap his energy.

Not only that, he must keep that energy going long enough for him and/or for his wife to climax. A very overweight person may struggle to have that level of stamina.

Obesity is often linked to poor heart health or arterial clogging, which can lessen blood flow. You know where a man needs blood flow for sex? Yep, that's right—his penis. Some men with unhealthy weight will struggle more with erectile dysfunction and thus sexual interest. Not being able to perform makes many husbands less likely to take the stage.

Another related health risk that can impact sexual desire and performance is type 2 diabetes, a common outcome of obesity. A small but interesting 2018 study compared men with prediabetes symptoms to nonsymptomatic men and concluded that prediabetic men showed disturbances in sexual desire.[2]

A Final Word on Proportion

In 2018, Michael Bublé made an appearance on *The Late Late Show* to sing carpool karaoke with host James Corden. When Corden asked Bublé about having lost a lot of weight, Bublé responded that he didn't care about his size, except that "when you're smaller, your penis looks bigger."[3]

Now, Bublé attested that his wife loved him regardless, but a lot of husbands are quite concerned about their penis size. If he doesn't feel like it's enough for his wife, he may, consciously or unconsciously, resist or be less enthusiastic about having sex.

If only I could get more husbands to understand that wives tend to believe their husbands are big enough, thank you very much. And whatever its size, she love his penis because it's part of the man she loves.

6. His Diet

"You are what you eat" is an idiom popularized by nutritionist Victor Lindlahr in the 1930s—the idea being that our health rests heavily on what we consume. Surely what we consume is not the whole of our identity, yet there's some truth to the notion that what we put into our bodies affects what our bodies can do. How might your husband's diet affect his libido and performance?

Conflicting Advice

When it comes to which foods experts say are good for us, the goalposts seem to keep moving. The recommended diets of yesteryear aren't necessarily on nutritionists' lists these days. In the case of the poached-egg-and-grapefruit diet my mother tried when I was young, thank goodness. We'll look at the best advice available today, but if something changes from what I share in this chapter, please don't send me hate mail with poop emojis. At least go with the sad-face emoji.

Foods That Ding His Drive

Some items on your husband's plate may be delicious but not ideal for sexual readiness. We're often not aware of the effect such foods can have on our health, especially on libido. But some choices can cause problems for a man's sexual desire. Here are a few culprits.

Sugar. So good and yet so bad. While it makes everything sweeter, if a guy overdoes the sugar, his testosterone could take a not-so-sweet dive. Studies in 2013 and 2018 showed that men experience a substantial decrease in T levels after consuming a large amount of sugar, which can last for hours.[1]

Even without research, we recognize that sugar causes energy spikes followed by crashes. Need proof? Give a kid cotton candy and wait. Now imagine that's your husband, and you can see why a diet high in sugar can leave him too pooped to pop.

We're not necessarily talking about candy and cake here. High-sugar foods include soda, juice, flavored coffees, canned soups, sauces, frozen meals, and boxed cereals. Basically, if there's an *-ose* in the ingredients—dextrose, fructose, etc.—the food contains sugar.

We're unlikely to avoid all sugar, but by avoiding high-sugar foods, your husband can consume a moderate amount that can help his overall health and sexual desire.

Carbohydrates. While sugars *are* carbohydrates, other foods also qualify—such as starches, which your body breaks down into sugar. In response, low-carb diets have become popular, and you or your husband may be tempted to try one out. But remember that a man needs some carbs for his body—and testosterone—to work properly.

It's not so much an issue of *how many* carbohydrates he should consume as *what kind*. Simple starches can result in those same sugar spikes and crashes, while complex starches are broken down over longer periods of time. What are simple starches? Examples include many of our favorites: white bread, white rice, potato chips, French fries, most pastas, flour tortillas (way to destroy this Tex-Mex enthusiast), and pastries.

Complex carbohydrates are our friends. Maybe not the friends we fully appreciate at the beginning, but the ones that have our backs, stomachs, or sex drive. Anyway, here are a few complex starches: pita bread, quinoa, potatoes, sweet potato fries, whole wheat pasta, corn tortillas (okay, I slightly forgive the dissing of my flour tortillas), and oats.

Swapping out simple for complex carbs is a good way to give your guy more energy and keep his body in shape.

Fat. The word "fat" has a terrible connotation, right? I grew up at a time when low-fat was all the rage among dietary experts, and they made it sound like a pat of butter once a week might summon an early heart attack.

But like simple versus complex carbohydrates, the reality is more complicated. There are bad fats and good fats. The former can add pounds to our bodies, bring plaque to our arteries, and sap sexual interest. So what are the bad fats?

Let's start with some good news. Artificial trans fats—the worst of the fats—have been banned in the European Union, the United States, and many other countries. If you're in one of those countries, you can't even get these fats, so you can relax and not worry about the worst offenders.

Now for the less-good news. Plenty of bad fats remain, and ooh, some of the foods they're in are delicious, such as fried foods, cookies, buttered popcorn, margarine, processed meats and cheeses, and many commercially manufactured snacks. But good fats are also delicious and can be found in nuts, salmon and tuna, olive oil, avocado, coconut, pasture-raised eggs, and grass-fed butter. These healthy options are most conducive to feeding a healthy sex drive.

God's Design for Our Diet

We've covered what experts say is good for living a healthy life. But what does God intend for us to eat? Consider the foods he mentions when describing the promised land in Deuteronomy 8:7–10:

> For the LORD your God is bringing you into a good land—a land with brooks, streams, and deep springs gushing out into the valleys and hills; a land with wheat and barley, vines and fig trees,

pomegranates, olive oil and honey; a land where bread will not be scarce. . . . When you have eaten and are satisfied, praise the LORD your God for the good land he has given you.

Apparently, God thought we could sate our appetite with grains, vegetables and fruits, and healthy fats. Of course, we know that God's people also ate meat and fish. What they didn't eat was a whole box of Girl Scout Thin Mints on a road trip to Tennessee. No, that would be me, circa 1991.

I doubt God is opposed to Thin Mints. No, they are a heaven-like cookie sold by green-vested angels. But we ought to consume healthy foods more often than indulgent ones, and not doing so can have an impact on our sex life.

How You Can Support Him

As you learn the importance of diet for sexual health, you may feel compelled to step away from this chapter, purge your fridge and pantry, and introduce a strict eating plan for your husband. But don't be his food police! It's not your job to monitor what goes on his plate or in his mouth. And taking that approach can make intimacy less likely to happen, because who wants to have sex with a dour diet detective? Remember, you're his *wife*, not his mother or probationary officer.

What you can do is inform your husband of what you've learned, make better choices when it's your turn to shop for groceries or cook a meal, and support his journey toward better health. Letting him know that his diet choices impact his sexual interest and performance might be just the thing to kickstart his own curiosity about what should go on his plate.

And if he wants or needs more direction, suggest that he consult his doctor, a dietitian, a nutritionist, or that one friend you have who reads all the health articles and books and would be more than happy to share. Just encourage him to avoid crash diets, which have their own negative impacts on physical health and sexual desire.

7. Alcohol and Drugs

From my favorite Shakespearean tragedy comes this line: "O God, that men should put an enemy in their mouths to steal away their brains! That we should, with joy, pleasance, revel, and applause, transform ourselves into beasts!"[1] The character, Cassio of *Othello*, is talking about getting drunk, but his sentiment applies to any substance that alters our perception.

Knocking Boots or Knocking Back?

Garth Brooks's popular song "Friends in Low Places" is mostly about drinking away your troubles, but too much whiskey and beer are enemies to a husband's "low places." Excessive alcohol consumption introduces more troubles into our lives, including in the bedroom.

As we all learned in health class many moons ago, alcohol is a depressant. It slows down the central nervous system—which translates to a person's perception, emotions, senses, and actions all being blunted. Note the impact on emotions and senses, both of which are extra important for pleasure and intimacy in the bedroom. If a man can't truly feel what's happening, he's missing out on how good the sex could be.

But that's assuming he makes it to the bedroom. Drinking too much also increases neurotransmitters that can make a person feel good without having sex but lead to fatigue, sleepiness, and nausea. No man in the fog of intoxication is at his sexual peak.

In addition, while men may be fans of beers and erections, if they have too much of the former, they aren't going to get many of the latter. Alcohol impairs blood flow in and out of the penis,[2] and the body prioritizes flushing alcohol from its system over maintaining an erection.

Heavy drinking can also dip one's testosterone while raising estrogen levels. For men, higher estrogen levels can sap libido, bring down mood, and make achieving orgasm more difficult.[3]

How much alcohol is too much? Recommendations vary, and your husband's size, tolerance, and background play into what counts as moderate or excessive. A healthcare professional could give a more tailored answer, but one resource to consult is "The Basics: Defining How Much Alcohol Is Too Much," an online article from the National Institute on Alcohol Abuse and Alcoholism.[4]

Can Cannabis Lead to Canoodling?

You may wonder why I'd even mention marijuana in a Christian book about sex. But at the time of this writing, twenty-four states have legalized recreational use, another twelve states allow medicinal use, and I've heard from several Christian couples who've added it to their lovemaking. Some have even shared with me peer-reviewed research indicating that marijuana can heighten sexual pleasure. So let's take a clear-eyed look at the evidence, and then we'll look at the issue through a biblical lens. (Spoiler: It fails on both counts.)

Researchers note that cannabis triggers the release of dopamine, giving the user euphoric feelings and possibly heightening sensory perception. But you know what else triggers the release of dopamine? Eating chocolate, kissing your lover, and exercise. What chemical substances typically do, however, is provide an unnatural spike of dopamine that ends with more of a crash, making the user yearn for the experience again. In fact, according to the National Institute on Drug Abuse, 30% of cannabis users may have some degree of marijuana use disorder, which typically means dependence.[5]

But, some argue, a 2017 study suggested that cannabis use is "associated with increased sexual frequency with daily and weekly users having significantly higher sexual frequency compared to never-users."[6] Given that lack of frequency is a common complaint for HDWs, could cannabis be part of the solution?

Not really. Much like a glass of wine can ease tension, so a small dose of marijuana can loosen things up for sexual engagement. But it's a crutch rather than a resolution, and it leads to other problems. Among them are a suppressed immune system, an increased heart rate, eye redness, increased risk of bronchitis (if marijuana is smoked), memory problems, slowed reaction times, and impaired judgment.[7] On top of all that, cannabis may lower sperm count and affect embryos fertilized from that sperm.[8]

Marnie shared with me her experience with her husband's marijuana use. Married later in life, she was optimistic and eager to engage in sexual intimacy. But over time, his cannabis use dampened his sexual interest: "He just doesn't notice when I try to drop hints and would rather get stoned and spend hours on end playing on his Xbox!" When her husband finally quit using marijuana, his sexual interest increased. Life situations that led to his use of it still needed to be addressed, but physiologically, his libido got a boost when he gave up pot.

If you're still thinking that marijuana might help your sex life, let's peer through that biblical lens. Having sex while under the influence is hardly what God designed sexual intimacy to be. Even if one accepts the idea that marijuana could at times be a shortcut to greater frequency and intensity, it robs couples of discovering and building true intimacy based on sober awareness and experience of one another.

Doing the Deed or Doping?

As I write this, there's a fentanyl crisis in the United States. According to the National Center of Health Statistics, a heartbreaking 106,000 people died from drug-involved overdose in 2021, and over 70,000 of those involved opioids, primarily fentanyl. Other drugs implicated include heroin, cocaine, and other prescription opioids.[9]

Death is obviously the worst consequence of drug abuse, but lesser drug use can hurt one's physical health, mental focus, sleep habits, and mood.[10] On top of all those issues—which certainly challenge a marriage—drug use can cause sexual dysfunction and lessened libido.

Opioids, cocaine, and amphetamines can appear to have positive sexual outcomes at first, providing users a heightened sense of arousal, decreased inhibition, and the ability to maintain an erection longer. But like the high itself, those "benefits" don't last. Rather, these drugs decrease testosterone and androgen, lower sexual desire, and cause erectile dysfunction.[11]

Even if mild doses of these drugs make sex more enjoyable short-term, they still rob the couple of being fully present and intimate. If a husband is using, it's time for him to get help and get clean. Only then can you assess what his true sexual function and desire are.

Remember These Cs

As much as I wish sharing this information meant you could go to your husband, show him the facts, and have a complete turnaround, that's not how this works. Alcohol and drug abuse isn't overcome in a moment, and the user may not be as motivated to change as you hope.

Alcohol and drug use can be hard to quit. Admitting the problem is a first step, but getting help is a difficult second step . . . and there are many steps after that.

How can you support your husband? Start by recognizing what you can't do.

Al-Anon, an organization for family members dealing with a loved one's alcoholism, teaches these three Cs:

1. I didn't cause it.
2. I can't control it.
3. I can't cure it.[12]

Remind yourself of these truths often.

But what can you do?

You can talk to your husband about your concerns and share what you've learned. You can practice self-care so that you're in a better mental and emotional space to deal with the struggles. You can look at whether you've unintentionally enabled his use and refrain from doing that in the future. You can set boundaries to protect yourself from being manipulated, used, or violated.[13] You can pray for your husband and for yourself.

While you cannot force your husband to stop using, you can make a difference. For help on this journey, check out Al-Anon, Nar-Anon, or other support groups for loved ones living with a user.

8. His Sleep

Plenty of folks blame Edison.

Thomas Alva Edison invented the electric light bulb, which made it possible for insomniacs, night owls, and overly busy people to stay up past dark—and not worry about the wick or the oil going out.

In our day, the culprit keeping us up is more likely the screen, represented by TV, tablets, and phones that give us access to information, entertainment, and connection 24/7. With so much activity at our fingertips, how do we shut it off long enough to get the good night's sleep we need?

And for those of you who are parents of young children, you don't need a light bulb or a screen. Your kids can make you more sleep-deprived than a Red Bull–fueled college student during finals week.

Lack of Sleep

We need sufficient sleep to have the energy to make love. But a lack of sleep can also affect a man's libido, sexual performance, and even sperm quality. Poor sleep correlates with lower levels of circulating testosterone and androgen, both of which play into sexual desire.[1] Insufficient sleep can also cause erectile difficulties.[2]

So when your husband is overly tired, his full sexual capacity is diminished—making him less likely to initiate or engage in sexual activity with you.

As for sperm quality, experts say that's not related to sexual desire, but if having kids is among your goals, you should know that the health of his swimmers is impacted by a lack of good sleep.

Excess Sleep

Now before you send your husband to bed for a twelve-hour nap, hoping he'll wake up with enough energy to go all night, let's talk about too much sleep.

Proverbs 6:9 asks, "How long will you lie there, you sluggard? When will you get up from your sleep?" The verses after warn that poverty comes to those who stay abed too much, too long. But it's not only a person's pocketbook that suffers. Sleeping too much can make it difficult for a man to achieve orgasm. And sexual performance difficulties tend to result in less sexual interest. After all, why take the stage if you know you're going to bomb? Or, in this case, fizzle out.

Goldilocks Sleep

"Moderation in all things." Although that saying is often presumed to come from the Bible, it's actually attributed to Greek poet Hesiod, who lived about seven hundred years before Christ.[3] The principle, however, is consistent with God providing what we need while warning against greed. For example, a worker is due his wages (Luke 10:7), but the rich man will struggle to enter the kingdom of God (Matt. 19:23). Likewise, we deserve our sleep, but not so much that we're ruled by sleep.

So what's that Goldilocks "just right" amount?

We need a regular routine with restorative sleep, especially rapid eye movement (REM) cycles—the stage of sleep when our mind is most active, when dreaming happens, and when our brains consolidate information. After he falls asleep, a man's testosterone levels rise, but then during the first REM cycle, they rapidly increase, and that cycle tends to happen about three hours in.[4] But a man needs well over three hours of sleep to maintain a healthy level of testosterone. One study showed a 10–15% decrease in testosterone levels for men restricted to five hours of sleep.[5]

Meanwhile, a research analysis of over 4,000 men showed that middle-aged men who got more than nine hours of sleep per night were more likely to have low testosterone levels than those who got seven to eight hours.[6]

Sleep experts, therefore, recommend seven to eight hours of sleep for most men, with one particular study showing better sexual health when men got at least seven and a half hours.[7] Still, what's right for your husband depends on his individual physiology.

Keeping similar bedtimes night to night and waking around the same time each day, seven and a half to nine hours later, may help both a husband's libido and his sexual performance.

Why Isn't He Sleeping?

Some times in life simply come with less sleep—tax season for accountants, the arrival of an infant for parents, Christmas services and walk-through Bethlehems for church leaders. But the rest of the time, we can and should pursue quality sleep. If that's not happening, start by asking why.

Among the reasons we struggle to fall asleep or to sleep well:

- having caffeine too close to bedtime
- staying on screens late at night
- eating supper too late
- bright light
- intrusive noise

- inconsistent bedtimes and wake times
- excessive alcohol consumption
- restless leg syndrome (an irresistible urge to move one's legs while trying to fall asleep)
- sleep apnea (disruptions to one's breath patterns during sleep)[8]

Those last two—restless leg syndrome and apnea—are sleep disorders that can be identified and treated by a sleep medicine specialist.[9] If your husband struggles to fall asleep, gets enough sleep but feels sleepy during the day, or falls asleep at unusual times, consult your healthcare provider to see if a sleep disorder might be the cause.

For other obstacles to sleeping well, here are a few tips:

- Do your best to maintain a consistent bedtime and wake time schedule.
- Avoid caffeine after midafternoon.
- Eat your last meal a couple of hours or more before bedtime.
- Turn off screens thirty minutes to an hour before bedtime.
- Create a wind-down routine that helps you relax.
- Lower the temperature in your bedroom (most people sleep best at sixty-five to sixty-eight degrees Fahrenheit).[10]
- Wear a sleep mask to block out light.
- Try sleep meditation music or sounds, especially those with binaural beats.
- Pray before you fall asleep, giving your worries to God and asking for his peace.

As Psalm 3:5 says, "I lie down and sleep; I wake again, because the LORD sustains me."

Now, remember that you cannot control all these for your husband! But where you can support his efforts to get better sleep, do so. And make sure you get enough sleep yourself; without it, you may be even more sensitive to his "not now" or "no" response to sexual initiation.

Sex Begets Better Sleep

One last thought on the relationship of sex and sleep: feeling sexually sated tends to help spouses sleep more soundly. You may have read this elsewhere and thought it was a good point to make to your husband: "Have sex with me, and we'll both sleep better!"

While true in the long term, it's not a great short-term bid. While I'm all about the physiological benefits of great sex in marriage, if your husband isn't that interested in sex, saying "do it for the sleep" isn't the right message to get him on board. You don't want sex to be on par with counting sheep.

If he's sleep-deprived, focus there first and then mention the sleep benefit of sex as he begins to experience more energy and interest.

9. Aging

While some wives have been the higher desire spouse throughout their marriage, many others enter their later years and discover their sexual interest has flipped. Where once *he* was the driven initiator, now *she* is the one eager to get to the bedroom. Some feel confused by this development, and others feel cheated because "he wanted it so much before, but when I want it, he doesn't care!"

Why did the mismatch flip? One reason is aging—for both of them.

First, let's look at you, higher desire wife, because that's part of the equation. Then we'll focus the rest of this chapter on an aging husband's sexuality.

How She Changed

Myriad reasons explain why a wife could have increased interest in sex later in life. Here are the most common ones.

Hormonal Changes. A woman's body goes through many changes during perimenopause, the yearslong transition time into menopause, which is defined as a point in time twelve months after a woman's last period. Two hormones that regulate ovulation, estrogen and progesterone, decrease. With the reduction of estrogen, the hormone testosterone is freer, so to speak, to have its day in the sun. Testosterone is definitely related to sex drive, and not being crowded out by other hormones needed for childbearing, it may assert itself with a newfound libido. Many wives report feeling randier in their forties, fifties, and beyond, and that's influenced by shifting hormones.

Leaving Motherhood. While raising children, women often experience mental and emotional stress, drains on physical energy, and time constraints that dampen their sexual interest. But when the kids are grown or nearly grown, some women find their fatigue lifts, their focus improves, and their interest in that good-lookin' guy they share a home with gets a big boost. Some wives even feel like this is their time to make up for those sacrificial years of active mommy duty and indulge in some sexy fun.

Improved Self-Image. In my age cohort (midfifties as of this writing), it's amazing how many of us feel worse about some aspects of our appearance yet so much better about our bodies and selves. With age often come the wisdom, maturity, and perspective that help us value who we are as a person more than how we measure up to unrealistic standards. Perhaps you relate to noticing how aging is taking a toll—with bags under your eyes; wrinkles here, there, and everywhere; more belly despite fewer calories; and breasts giving in to gravity—but also to feeling more confident in your own skin and happy with who you are. Given that our husbands have their own aging issues, the appearance aspect doesn't matter nearly as much as "Hey, I feel good about myself—let's get naked!"

Negative Self-Image. After reading the reason right above this one, you think, *Wait a minute.* Yet while some wives feel more confident, other wives struggle with the wear and tear of life on their bodies. Previously, the wife who felt good about how she looked now wonders, "Can he really be attracted to this version of me?" Then she tests it out by pursuing more sex, hoping to calm the anxiety in her heart and make herself feel sexy and beautiful again.

Cracking the Code. Arousal, foreplay, positions, orgasm . . . The various aspects of sexual engagement can be difficult to figure out, and only later in life do some women "crack the code" of their sexuality. Suddenly, it seems, they've figured out what works—especially orgasm—and not surprisingly, they're eager to take advantage of their new expertise. They might even be excited to show off what they can do for their husbands as well, now that they've got the skillz. (Yes, that's skills with a *z*. Look it up, fellow aging lady! [wink])

Whatever your reason for being more interested in sex, your "let's get this party started" attitude may be met with an aging husband's desire to skip the party and go to bed early. To sleep. Why is that?

Speaking of Testosterone

In chapter 4, we talked about how low testosterone can lower male sex drive, and that can happen as men get older. Our primary sex hormones decrease as we age—estrogen for us gals and testosterone for the guys. According to Harvard Health,

> In some men, testosterone levels remain high throughout life, but in most they begin to decline at about age 40. Unlike the precipitous drop in hormones that women experience at menopause, however, the decline in men is gradual, averaging just over 1% a year. This drop is imperceptible at first, but by age 70, the average man's testosterone production is 30% below its peak.[1]

What men experiencing this decline have told me is they simply don't have the same sense of urgency to their sex drive. Far more often, they could take sex or leave it. And while they might have happily skipped sleep before, they find themselves weighing the two and not sure which way to go. It can be a confusing time for those gents, especially when on top of their own wondering what's wrong with them, their wife is wondering too.

Gail struggled to want and enjoy sex earlier in her marriage, but when she realized that her resistance had deeply hurt her husband, she took steps to change. As she was working through the reasons why she'd been less interested, her hormones shifted and her kids grew up. All that put together resulted in a fresh discovery of desire. But once she became more than eager to engage, her husband's sexual peak had passed: "So he gets into his sixties, and he's fine with twice a week. He would have been happy to have acknowledged or participated if I would have initiated, but I wanted him to want me. I wanted him to be the one."

Gail's drive was increasing as her husband's was decreasing, and the match in sexual interest seemed to last but a moment. Gone too soon.

One way in which this experience of lower desire is different for men is when they've tied their sense of masculinity to that testosterone-driven appetite. They might feel even worse if they're reminded by their eager-for-sex wife that they can't keep up. To protect his sense of self and heart, a man might shun sex more than he actually wants to, because he hates facing what he fears— that his best days are over.

You and I know there are many good days left, but take a minute to feel compassion for these men who haven't gone through vast hormonal changes since adolescence—and that change felt like becoming a man. This one feels quite different.

Bones, Muscles, and Joints, Oh My!

You know what else breaks down as you age? Everything. Including the bones, muscles, and joints used during sex. And let's face it, ladies: unless you're on top or giving him oral sex, he's likely exerting more physical effort than you are. Your husband may be balancing his desire for sex with his desire to do it without pain or simply the way he used to do it.

An aging husband may not be able to get into the same positions, maintain them as long, or thrust as hard. Moreover, an aching back, hips, or knees can be distracting or at least lower the amount of satisfaction he gets from sex. He might power through, but he might also turn down opportunities because he doesn't feel quite up to it.

Problems of the Prostate

Another part of a man's body that can affect sexual desire is the prostate. The prostate is a rubbery gland smaller than a golf ball and deeply positioned between the base of a man's penis and his rectum. Its reproductive role is to coordinate with the seminal vesicles to produce semen, and manual massage of the prostate (internally or externally) can provide pleasurable sensations.

Most men experience an enlarged prostate as they age. Known as benign prostatic hyperplasia (BPH), this condition affects about 50% of men over age 60 and 85% of men over age 80.[2] What does that mean for sex?

Not much, unless he gets treatment for an enlarged prostate. And healthcare providers suggest treatment when it interferes with urination. Over half of men with BPH don't have symptoms,[3] but those who do can experience the following:

- an urgent need to urinate and difficulty postponing urination
- a hesitation before urine flow starts despite the urgency to urinate
- straining when urinating
- weak or intermittent urinary stream
- a sense that the bladder has not emptied completely
- dribbling at the end of urination or leakage afterward
- a frequent need to awaken from sleep to urinate

Well, that sounds unpleasant. So of course a guy going through that would want something to make it stop!

Treatments involve everything from lifestyle changes to medications to surgical intervention. Unfortunately, the latter two treatments could cause temporary or permanent ejaculatory problems, making it harder for him to complete a sexual encounter. Indeed, dry orgasm—spasms without a release of semen—can happen occasionally or regularly. Dry orgasm can still be satisfying, but it feels different. For some men, the climax is stronger, but for others, it's weaker.[4] Such struggles with ejaculation are not the pleasant experience a man desires during sex with his wife, but they're likely preferable to the discomfort and leakage they'd have during urination without treatment.

If this is an issue, recognize that his climax may be delayed and may require more direct stimulation. That could involve changing sexual positions to increase friction on his penis, using his or your hand to finish, or adding a marital aid to your touch, such as a small bullet or fingertip vibrator, which you can purchase through an online Christian retailer.[5] Also, timing sex according to his medication schedule can help—that is, gauging when the medication is at its lowest effect during the day and making love near that time.

Not Pumping Like It Used To

Another (annoying) result of getting older is decreased blood flow. You know how our bodies become less pliable and stiffer as we age? That's happening inside us too—with our heart walls and valves, arteries and veins. All of which come down to our blood not pumping quite as efficiently as it did when we were young.

The penis needs only a few ounces of blood to become erect, but not getting all it needs makes the erection less hard. The blood flow might still get there but take more time and require more stimulation. This change in his tumescence (the cool scientific word for blood swelling his penis) can be disappointing, frustrating, or confidence sapping for some husbands.

If your husband experiences erectile dysfunction, it could be due to lessened blood flow. To find answers, he should start by seeing a healthcare practitioner. While less-hard erections are typical for aging, they can also indicate other health problems, such as diabetes or cardiovascular disease. His penis's less-than-rigid lift could be a red flag for a more dire condition, one you shouldn't ignore.

I'm sure you believe a noncooperative penis is a somewhat dire situation in and of itself. I bet your husband sees it that way too. And for men who shrug it off and say that's just what happens as you age, I suspect they also care but don't know what to do about it and don't want to dwell on what they cannot fix.

Reassure your guy that yes, aging impacts penile firmness, but it's not a death knell for his love muscle. Greater stimulation to the area can increase blood flow, and we can assist our bodies' blood flow overall through moderate exercise, healthy eating, and not smoking. Suggest regular romantic walks to get you both in shape, and it might help things swell better where and how they should.

Although the quantity and intensity of sexual encounters can diminish as we age, many older couples report the quality of sexual intimacy is better than ever. They view these challenges as an opportunity to learn new ways of being sexual, to serve one another more fully, and to savor the slower pace of lovemaking. It can take time to find a new rhythm, but if you do, you might say to one another, as poet Robert Browning put it, "Grow old along with me! The best is yet to be."[6]

10. Chronic Disease or Illness

If your husband has a chronic disease or illness, you likely know it. Whether it's diabetes, multiple sclerosis, fibromyalgia, cancer, or another chronic condition, you may recognize the illness and/or treatment are responsible for your husband's lack of libido or sexual dysfunction.

But that doesn't mean you're okay with it. You might be positive and patient most of the time, but now and then, you wonder why it has to be so difficult. And perhaps why your husband doesn't seem as disappointed with the lack of sex as you are.

One More Thing

One of my favorite *Saturday Night Live* characters ever was Roseanne Roseannadanna, a consumer affairs reporter played by Gilda Radner who had the irritating habit of going off topic to rant about personal hygiene or bodily functions. When asked what her tangent had to do with the original subject, she'd always respond, "Well, it just goes to show you, it's always something—if it's not one thing, it's another."

Someone with chronic illness can feel like that when lack of sex gets brought up. Yes, your husband recognizes sex is missing, but with his focus taken up by his overall health, the sex issue feels like one more thing he can't control. He may simply shut down in that area, not wanting to be reminded of one more failure of his body.

Of course, you don't see it that way. You find him sexually attractive and well worth the effort to overcome challenges. But a lot of this book is about putting yourself in your husband's shoes to try to understand and empathize with where he's coming from. If he feels your support, he's more likely to be willing to discuss the missing pieces of your marital intimacy.

Be gentle with how you bring up your concerns, letting him know you're not trying to add one more burden but rather remove an obstacle to enjoying your life together.

Balancing the Battle

Most people with chronic disease feel they're in a balancing act. They want enough treatment to stop the progression or impact of the disease while not introducing more side effects than they can withstand. One side effect of many medications is decreased sex drive, and other medications can cause sexual dysfunction. But they need that treatment more than they need sex. So much for balance!

Many times, however, adjustments can be made to rebalance the equation—*if* the doctor knows about it. A healthcare professional can't do anything about a problem they're unaware of.

Encourage your husband to ask questions about sexual health and treatment alternatives. Offer to come to the appointments with him so you can hear for yourself what's possible and not possible—and thus live more peacefully with the outcome.

Pursuing Intimacy over Intercourse

Let your husband know what you actually want. When asked about sex, he may feel that he needs to participate at full energy, when you might be fine with an encounter far short of that. After all, feeling desired and intimate outweigh "git 'er done."

Talk about what your sexual repertoire can entail, given the challenges he faces. If he can't achieve an erection, would he be willing to make out, provide you manual stimulation, caress you while you bring yourself to climax, or just naked-cuddle for a while? Is there something that would make him feel sexually known and loved? Should you add a tool to make sexual encounters easier, such as a bullet vibrator, penis ring, wedge pillow, or other marital aid? Such sex toys may be off-putting for some, but couples with particular health challenges may benefit from well-chosen aids that alleviate obstacles to sexual enjoyment and satisfaction.

Discuss the importance of rain checks when he's not up to engaging. You'll feel much better getting that "no" if it comes with a promise that you two can be sexual later, when he's up to it. Depending on your circumstances, that could mean later in the day, the following day, or within the next week. A rain check isn't a guarantee, but it's a promise to try again. Creating the habit of rain checks can reaffirm the importance of sex to both of you.

Make it clear that intimacy is your goal, and sex is one avenue—an important one, but not the only one—for pursuing that end.

Frustrating Flare-Ups

Even if you can address sexual intimacy better, you'll have frustrating moments—times when a flare-up or disease progression makes you grieve yet again what's been lost. And as much as you don't want to, you can feel resentment. Why has this illness targeted your marriage? Why doesn't your husband take better care of himself or pursue better treatments? Why must you, a healthy wife, go without sex again and again?

My husband has had type 1 insulin-dependent diabetes for forty-five years, including all thirty-two years of our marriage. When he was younger, we rarely had to skip a sexual encounter, but type 1 diabetes progresses, and in later years we've experienced more challenges to our lovemaking. Usually it's about timing, when high or low blood sugar prevents him from engaging in a particular moment. But sometimes the overall impact of the disease makes him not feel as good as he would otherwise. And his diabetes is well controlled.

I'd be lying if I said I haven't felt cheated at times. I'm not upset with him, but I am upset at the situation—the unfairness of it, the missed opportunities for physical and emotional intimacy. I become weary of getting my hopes up only to be told "I can't" because his body isn't cooperating.

How can you manage those letdowns? Again, if your husband already feels bad, let's not heap more guilt on the man. He didn't choose that disease. A broken world did it for him. He's likely already aware of your disappointment, and hearing your frustration may feel like pressure rather than motivation.

Go ahead and grieve! This stinks. For both of you. But look for safe spaces to lament: to a counselor, a trusted mentor, a marriage-positive friend, your loving heavenly Father. Feel the feelings, but then remember the goal.

Consider how you'll respond to those inevitable moments. What self-talk can help you get through the disappointment? What other ways can you pursue intimacy with your husband? Do you see other signs that he loves and desires you outside of sexual passion? What part can you play in helping him manage his illness or disease? Answer these questions ahead of time so you're prepared when a frustrating flare-up and subsequent brush-off come your way.

Then put into practice some of the tips laid out in this chapter, as well as the real-life advice in the "Now What?" part later in the book. Neither of you wanted this challenge, but you can tackle it together.

11. Ongoing Pain

I have a friend who's in a sexless marriage. Her husband has had severe back problems for years, and the pain and discomfort make it difficult, at best, for him to engage in sex. They've prioritized other ways to be intimate, but it would be better for them and their marriage if his back problems could be resolved. Thankfully, they're pursuing just that—treatments to address the underlying cause of pain.

Body Hurts

Perhaps your husband has pain or discomfort that makes sexual encounters a challenge. Even if sex is possible, his pleasure is diminished by aches or strains that make lovemaking less enjoyable. In the long run, that makes the whole kit and caboodle less appealing. He may want sex with his wife, but does he want the pain that comes with it?

If you know pain is your husband's issue, of course you want him to deal with it. Unfortunately, some men don't seek medical help when they need it, for reasons from hoping it will go away to not wanting to spend money on healthcare. Your best approach may be to remind your husband that his health matters to you—not just in the bedroom but well beyond. Help him figure out how he can find time in his schedule, money in your budget, or assistance to get his must-dos done during treatment or recovery.

If he has tried treatment that didn't work, ask him to try again. Another doctor may conduct different tests or have a different perspective, or new approaches may have been introduced since he sought help. Here's one possible analogy to use with your husband: Assume you take a misbehaving car to a mechanic, but the shop doesn't fix it. You likely wouldn't just say, "Oh well, it's broken." You'd take it back and insist they try again or take it to a different mechanic and see what they can do. Surely we should treat our bodies as well as we treat our cars.

But it's also possible that your husband simply isn't telling you about his pain, believing "it's not that bad" or he can grit his way through it. He may be unaware of how the pain or discomfort has impacted his sexual interest. Even if you don't think this is an issue, it might be worth discussing with one another any physical challenges you have during sex.

For instance, when I share that sometimes my hip gets stiff and makes certain sexual positions unpleasant, my husband feels freer to share that his knees hurt in other positions. (Hey, we're getting old. It happens.)

Sexual Pain

In addition to pains in the rest of his body, a man can experience pain in his genitalia. A bladder or yeast infection can make sex uncomfortable. Yes, men can get bladder and yeast infections too. A herpes infection or other sore on his penis can cause discomfort (and if that happens, you should refrain during an outbreak or use a condom). Small tears or lacerations in the skin can create sensitivity and pain. A prolonged erection, typically defined as one that lasts four or more hours, can be uncomfortable and cause difficulty with orgasm.[1]

Then there are penis anomalies, such as a tight foreskin (in uncircumcised men) or Peyronie's disease, which causes curved, painful erections.[2] And a few men react negatively to vaginal fluids or birth control methods, like having an allergy to latex condoms.[3]

While it may be tempting for him or you to believe he can push past the pain, that's a bad idea. Connecting sex with pain can be traumatic or disheartening and lead to dissociation or resentment. And no one—man or woman—should be expected to put up with pain during sex. That's not how God designed this intimate act.

All of the issues mentioned above can be medically addressed. If your husband has ongoing pain in his genitalia or testicular swelling, he should see a doctor. While some conditions have easy treatments, others could signal a significant health problem (for example, testicular cancer) that must be addressed quickly and thoroughly for the sake of his overall health.

Encourage your husband to take his sexual pain seriously and seek help to get answers.

Handle with Care

Finally, there's the possibility that you're not handling his goods gently enough. Those testicles in particular can be fragile. He may not have the heart to tell you that you're too rough, especially if he believes he's too sensitive or it doesn't hurt that much and he (erroneously) thinks he can get past it.

Ask your husband what his touch preferences are. What kind of strokes feel good? What about pressure and friction? Ask him to teach you what he likes and even to cover your hand with his to guide you until he can relax and enjoy what's happening.

Attending to your husband's sensitivities and addressing his pain or discomfort can make sex more enjoyable for both of you and more appealing for him.

PERSONAL HISTORY

"What's past is prologue" is engraved on a sculpture outside the National Archives building in Washington, DC. But the sculptor didn't think up that phrase. It's a quote from Shakespeare's *The Tempest*.[1]

But what a perfect way to say what we all know: our personal histories influence who we are today. We cannot escape the past, but we can recognize where it put us on a good path and where it diverted us. We can face difficult memories, learn, and find ways to heal. We can let God's resurrection power and the wise counsel of others renew our hearts, minds, and souls.

In this section, we'll talk about how the past has impacted your husband and how to take hold of a better future.

12. Poor Modeling

Heather was raised by "kinda hippie" parents who didn't shy away from the topic of sex, but her husband experienced a far different upbringing. Almost all of his sex education involved living on a farm and watching animals. As for his parents, Heather said, "They never ever talked about it. Sex was not something that was brought up. He didn't have any sex ed in school either because that wasn't a thing at the time."

Heather was surprised when they didn't have sex on their wedding night. She chalked it up to him being tired or wanting to take it slow, but his disinterest continued. Even though sex is fantastic when they have it, he seems uncomfortable pursuing it. His parents' silence likely played into his reticence regarding sexual intimacy.

The Seemingly Celibate Parents

Many kids grow up not only believing their parents don't have sex but also having little to no example of romance, affection, and intimacy from them. Perhaps your husband was one of them.

He may be right, with his mom and dad (or stepparent or partner) existing more as roommates or household comanagers than friends and lovers. Or maybe he had parents who hid their touching behind closed doors, as if any display of affection would be inappropriate for others' eyes.

But whatever the reality, his parents seemed celibate. A child raised in this atmosphere may view his parents' model as "the way it is" or "the way it should be." He could have a vague sense that marriage is where sex goes to die and that only the honeymoon years involve a lot of lovemaking. After that, it's down to the business of life, such as work and parenting.

The Sexually Explicit Parents

On the other hand, some husbands and wives have fuzzy boundaries about their sex life, and their children grow up knowing maybe more than they should. If adults take no steps to maintain privacy, appear in various states of undress or highly sexualized attire, or share details about their sex life, that can make a child feel awkward and even unsafe.

When that kid grows up, he may struggle to relax and enjoy touching, flirting, and lovemaking, because he doesn't want to be like *them*. His understandable desire to forge a different path can unconsciously sap his sexual desire and comfort.

The Super Silent Parents

Have you ever been around someone who cannot say the word "sex"? Perhaps they whisper it, spell it out, or only use euphemisms like "marital union," "consummation," "intimacy," or "you know" with an IYKWIM side glance. Perhaps they refuse to speak of it at all, shutting down any reference to sex because they believe it's not for Christians to talk about such things.

Those people might want to open up their Bible and see how honest God and his people were about sexuality! But my bigger point is that some husbands were raised by parents who didn't and even couldn't speak about sex. Sex was a taboo subject that at best received hushed tones and may have instead been relegated to the likes of "we don't talk about Bruno."[1]

While some men shirk off these constraints later in life, others absorb this tension about sex. Is it okay to talk about? To engage in? To enjoy? And what if something doesn't go as expected? If it can't be talked about, it can't be resolved . . . but again, it can't be talked about. What was modeled to this husband was basically one big *shhhhhh!*

The Adult Child

All parents mess up in some way or another. But while we can't reach perfection, the Christian community as a whole could do much better. Specifically, churches and family resources should (1) help parents do a better job preparing their children to understand God's design for sexuality, and (2) help adult children of parents who *didn't* do that well to embrace God's design for sexuality. You may need to help your husband identify the poor modeling he received—without insulting his parents, please. Simply talk about what you each learned about sex growing up and how it impacted your perspective.

If your husband struggles to have that conversation, try sharing your own story first and letting him chew on it before his turn. Also, note that many men feel more comfortable with shoulder-to-shoulder conversations than face-to-face ones, so perhaps bring up the subject while on a walk or drive somewhere. Written communication is also an option; I've had a lot of good "conversations" with my husband by emailing him an article I read, asking his opinion, and then messaging back and forth.

Invite your husband to come up with his own view of sexuality based on God's design and what seems healthier than what was taught or modeled to him in the past. For instance, you could ask a straightforward question like "How would you like our sexual intimacy to be different from the way our parents handled it in their marriage?" Sometimes speaking aloud how a person *wishes* it could be can set the stage for the next step and the next and the next.

However you address this, show compassion. We were formed in childhood, and we often still carry wounds, big and small, from those tender years. You don't want to trigger trauma or come across as attacking him or his family; rather, acknowledge how some teaching and modeling may have gotten in the way of healthy sexual intimacy, and determine how you can make progress.

13. Purity Messaging

For too long and in too many churches, sex has been addressed like it's a bad thing. It's either improper to discuss the topic or the focus is almost entirely on sexual sin. Instead of leaders sharing how God's gift of sexuality is something to both appreciate and manage well, they conveyed so many warnings that sex itself feels dangerous.

When kids and teens grow up hearing that sex is like a fire that could permanently burn you if mishandled in the slightest way, they behave like kids and teens do. One kid tests how close they can get to the fire without getting burned, another teases the fire with both curiosity and caution, and yet another stands far back with panic repressing their interest.

Yes, the analogy that sex is like a fire, which can wound if not controlled yet is a source of warmth if kept in the fireplace where it belongs, can help us understand that sex belongs in marriage. But the message of "Danger! Danger!" must be balanced with a full understanding of God's gift of sex. And the church has fallen short on that end of the scale.

"Purity culture" refers to an evangelical movement that reached its height in the late 1990s and early 2000s. It encouraged and cajoled teens and singles to stay "pure" (that is, maintain virginity) by saying no to dating, pursuing courtship instead, holding off on physical affection until well into the relationship, and taking purity pledges.[1]

While I didn't grow up with purity culture per se, the "don't have sex" message was prevalent. Maintaining your virginity was a mark of being a good Christian, and if you crossed that line, you could repent and behave better but could never get back the purity you once had. Losing your virginity was like losing a sock in the dryer—now in the lost and never-to-be found.

To put it plainly, for too many Christians, virginity became an idol.

Women Aren't the Only Ones

In the last decade or so, many Christian women have described the damage the purity message wrought in their lives. Women who embraced the purity message often disliked their own bodies, bore enormous guilt not only for sinful actions but also for temptation and normal sexual feelings, and couldn't allow themselves to experience or enjoy sex in marriage. In books, articles, videos, and more, female Christian leaders have challenged the unbiblical aspects of the purity message and called for a fresh vision more consistent with God's Word. It's a positive development that we're addressing these issues head-on and encouraging women to adopt a better understanding of God's design for sex.

But men heard a lot of these messages too. Many of them, fearful their sexual desire made them bad or less than, repressed their sexuality. And that two-ton weight of worry before the wedding vows got dragged into marriage.

In *The Language of Sex*, author and pastor Ted Cunningham shares about his own difficulty flipping the switch: "Sex was a shame-based teaching while I was growing up. I was not equipped to deal with or think properly about sex. The belief that started to be developed in my heart was subtle. For some reason I felt like a pervert when I initiated sex with my wife."[2]

He was several years into marriage before his wife pointed out that she initiated sex nine times out of ten. I can only imagine what she felt before that confession. Thankfully, this wise wife found the courage to bring up the topic, the compassion to listen to her husband's struggles, and the commitment along with him to change their sexual script.

Problematic Purity Messages

Most teachers who promoted purity messages were well-intentioned, wanting to spare young people the heartbreak and real-world consequences of sexual immorality. Indeed, Christians should continue to promote abstinence before marriage, since God clearly outlines it in Scripture as the ideal.

But we shouldn't end the message there or scare young people so much that they believe sexual misdeeds are in the category of unforgivable sin. The God whose mercy is great and who has removed our wrongdoings "as far as the east is from the west" (Ps. 103:12) stands ready to forgive and wipe the slate clean. Moreover, the Bible has a lot of good things to say about sex—from how "made in his image" includes our sexuality, whether we're single or married, to how God created sex not only for reproduction but also to strengthen the marital bond—and such messages need to be prominently shared.

Yet some husbands have a low libido or don't act on their sexual desire because they have learned to repress their sexuality based on purity myths. Which myths did they unwittingly embrace? See if any of these sound familiar:

- Not having sex makes you godlier.
- A woman wearing clothes that display her shape or skin is tempting you to look at her sexually.
- When you notice a pretty woman, you should bounce your eyes away from her to avoid lust.

- Men are naturally given to lust and/or struggle with pornography and will never gain victory over those temptations.
- Physical touch and kissing while dating or engaged are problematic, because they could awaken sexual interest.

You may not realize the impact such messages had on your husband and how they led to sexual repression. He may not consciously understand their influence in creating tension around his sexual feelings or his unwillingness to let himself "go there." The very definition of *repression* is "the process and effect of keeping particular thoughts and wishes *out of your conscious mind* in order to defend or protect it."[3]

Adding Shame to Guilt

To avoid sin, a man may inadvertently repress his sexuality. Maybe he keeps it bottled up and sealed tightly so he doesn't have to contend with the struggle. But maybe it leaks out from time to time through lustful thoughts, a brief but deep dive into pornography, or a make-out session gone too far—all of which serve to convince him once again how dangerous his sexuality is.

When a man who repressed his sexuality to remain "pure" enters marriage, more purity culture messages come into play, such as:

- Husbands want sex more than their wives.
- If you wait until marriage, sex will be effortless and wonderful.
- Men who don't have a strong drive toward sex are lying to themselves about their sexuality or are not real men.

Instead of tangling with guilt, as he did before marriage, a husband with a low sex drive may feel shame. His wife wants sex more than he does, meaning he cannot satisfy her the way he thought he would. Sex is not effortless and wonderful for him. Moreover, what does this mean about his identity as a man? What is so deeply wrong with him that he doesn't want sex all the time?

In the company of other men, such a man may fake it—pretending he is, in fact, the higher drive spouse. Why? Because he doesn't need more shame heaped on him from the brotherhood. He feels enough self-doubt and anxiety all on his own.

How much of this is within a husband's awareness? Probably not much. Some are more aware than others, but a fair number don't recognize the role purity themes have played in their inability to engage with sexual freedom in marriage.

Recovering from Repression

How can you help your husband move from repression to randiness? Acknowledge that problematic purity messages created misunderstandings about sex.

This doesn't mean your husband will one day spill the story of how all the teaching about purity he gathered while growing up cut him off from his true sexual self and how he longs for a better, godlier way. Most of us come to recognition over time, as we reveal ourselves slowly in a safe atmosphere with another. This is one reason why prayer can be so important—it's the ultimate safe atmosphere to share our struggles and concerns with God. But marriage should be another safe place to be known, accepted, and supported.

Begin the conversation about what you each learned about sex growing up. Share your own experiences with purity teaching and then ask him questions. What was it like when he became aware of his sexuality? How did he feel about spontaneous or reactionary erections? What teaching about sex from his parents, youth group, or other sources stuck with him? How does he think those impacted his expectations about sex in marriage? What does he wish he'd known before he got married?

These questions are examples for getting the conversation started. And by conversation, I mean *conversations*, plural. If it took years to build that wall between your husband and his natural sexual interest in a woman he loves, then it will take some time to pull it down.

Yes, I know sometimes we'd rather bulldoze that wall. But we don't want to injure our husband's heart, so we must take a more surgical approach to remove the barriers and keep the relationship intact.

Remind yourself and him that purity doesn't come from what we do or don't do but from God's purification of us through Jesus Christ's sacrifice. We are pure because of him, and our lives demonstrate that grace and God's blessing of our marriage with beautiful sexual intimacy with our spouse.

14. Prior Relationships

God's initial plan was one woman and one man united in marriage, followed by uniting in sex. While ancient weddings did not look like ours, Scripture consistently shows the righteous pattern to be one of covenant before copulation.

How many Christians meet that ideal? After looking for statistics on what percentage of Christians have premarital sex, I can honestly say that I don't know. That's because it matters how you define Christian (self-identified or practicing), the participation rate in some studies was problematic, and a lot of the data focuses on young people. But every source estimated the number at 65% or higher. So yeah, a hefty majority of us didn't get to our wedding night as the lily-white virgins some expected us to be.

And that's okay. I mean, it's not perfect. I definitely didn't reach the altar with my "V card" intact and experienced hurtful consequences of my promiscuity. But I later experienced God's deep compassion and full redemption. Please believe me when I say that if you or your husband had premarital sex, God is not holding that over you.

> For as high as the heavens are above the earth,
>   so great is his love for those who fear him;
> as far as the east is from the west,
>   so far has he removed our transgressions from us.
>   (Ps. 103:11–12)

God not only offers forgiveness, healing, and redemption in his love and compassion, but he longs for us to be satisfied with the things he created for us to enjoy (Ps. 103:2–5), including marital sex.

That said, having prior sexual relationships can impact our view of ourselves, sexuality, and sexual intimacy, even in the holy context of marriage. After all, God's design of sex between husband and wife has never been about keeping us from the goodies; rather, it places proper boundaries around sex so we can enjoy it fully in a safe space. When we don't follow that plan, we can get hurt.

Bringing in Shame

For years after I got married, I struggled with viewing my high interest in sex with my husband as a continuation of premarital promiscuity. Sure, it was legit now, but maybe I still deserved the "slut" label. Yes, sadly, that's the word that ran through my mind.

Some spouses enter marriage with deep shame about what they did in prior relationships. Despite being in the God-approved relationship of marriage, a shame-filled husband may carry guilt about wanting sex. He may feel bad about certain sexual activities he did and even worse if he still desires those activities. He may have defined himself as a sexual scoundrel, given how he treated women with whom he had brief interactions or one-night stands. He doesn't trust his sexuality, so he suppresses his sexual interest.

He may do so consciously, aware he's shutting things down to avoid more shame. But more likely, this suppression happens at a subconscious level, with him not feeling as interested in sex as he used to be.

A higher desire wife married to a husband like this laments that he had all kinds of sex with other women, so why won't he have sex with her? The irony is that it's often his deep love for his wife that keeps him from treating her like he did other women. He holds himself to a higher standard with her, because his love for her sets a higher standard for him.

88

The only way for him to get past such shame is to embrace the forgiveness, healing, and redemption God offers and to recognize that, regardless of what he did before, God longs to bless him now. If God can get past the sins of Moses, David, and Paul to use them mightily for his kingdom, he can and will redeem your husband's sexuality and renew him in his love.

Easier said than done. It took me many months of processing through the guilt I'd internalized, crying out to God, and replacing negative self-talk with God's truths to fully *feel* "there is now no condemnation for those who are in Christ Jesus" (Rom. 8:1).

If you think your husband is dealing with this struggle, I'd encourage you to go through some excellent resources about God and sexuality with your husband, such as my book *Hot, Holy, and Humorous: Sex in Marriage by God's Design*, Juli Slattery's *God, Sex, and Your Marriage*, or Joshua Ryan Butler's *Beautiful Union*. We all believe in the healing power of Christ in our areas of sexual brokenness, and hearing that message could show your husband the need to let go of the past and embrace God's steadfast love.

> The steadfast love of the LORD never ceases;
>   his mercies never come to an end;
> they are new every morning;
>   great is your faithfulness. (Lam. 3:22–23 ESV)

Getting Burned

Maybe your husband doesn't have lingering shame about previous sexual encounters, but sex was a sore spot in prior relationships. And his feelings about that have carried over into your marriage.

Imagine if your guy went through something like this with an earlier sexual partner:

- She said his penis wasn't big enough to satisfy her.
- She called him a pervert for wanting sex or a particular activity, one that was fairly mainstream.
- She cheated on him.
- She turned him down sexually over and over.
- She used sex as a weapon, denying it to him when she felt he'd misbehaved.
- She used sex as a reward, giving it to him when she felt he'd behaved well.

I've heard all of those stories, some several times. And such experiences can leave a mark on a husband's heart and mind. Generally speaking, each of them creates a feeling that sex is emotionally risky. He doesn't feel safe enough about himself or with you—despite you being in a different category—to experience sexual freedom.

Again, it could be conscious or subconscious, but his sex drive got dampened by him being burned. If only it had been just you and him in a garden like Adam and Eve in Eden! But don't entertain that notion for too long, because that's no one's story after Genesis 2. We all come into marriage with some sexual brokenness, and God knows and can work with where we are.

If you believe prior relationships negatively impacted your husband's sexual interest, get curious. Not critical. Not pushy. But inquisitive. Start by sharing your own sexual history—where you learned about sex, what you gleaned about sex from prior relationships, and what painful feelings and erroneous scripts followed you. Then ask him to share the same. Not to make this chapter a shameless plug for my books, but *Pillow Talk: 40 Conversations About Sex for Married Couples* helps couples have tough but enlightening conversations like these. Whether you grab a resource like mine or not, launch the conversation with gentle questions and a willingness to really listen and try to understand.

Once we pull back the curtain on what messages about ourselves and sex we absorbed from prior experiences, we can begin to address those messages with grace, truth, and love. Your reassurance may be key in this process as you let your beloved husband know that you chose him, you desire him, and you're there for him while he works through the pain of his past.

Compartmentalizing Sex

One of my greatest achievements was teaching my now-grown sons that marriage is not where sex falls off a cliff, Wile E. Coyote style. *Splat*. Rather, marriage is where the best sex can happen and thrive—it's the Road Runner of sex, if you will.

Not everyone believes that. Too many buy into the idea that one sows their wild oats before marriage, then settles down to a more serious existence after the wedding. Sex was fun before, but now that it's paired with partnering through life, it's not as exciting. Of course, that's a self-fulfilling prophecy—an expectation that something will happen that leads you to make it happen through your own (often unconscious) behaviors. So if a husband believes sex won't be as good in marriage, he may not pursue it with the same fervor he did in prior relationships. He may view it as an obligation more than a pleasurable act. He may become less interested in sex overall because "it won't be the same."

Of course it won't be the same, dude. It should be better!

Our minds have powerful sway over our feelings and actions. We must change our underlying beliefs to take hold of the first-class sexual intimacy we can have in marriage. If he's compartmentalized sex as being the best in his premarriage "glory days," he may unwittingly set himself up for a ho-hum experience in marriage—even though that's where God's Word tells husband and wife to "drink your fill of love" (Song of Songs 5:1).[1]

A husband in this situation needs to adjust his expectations to align with God's design and desire to bless Christian marriages with beautiful sexual intimacy. Discussing together your expectations and beliefs about sex pre- and post-marriage might open up a healthy conversation and an opportunity to pursue what the Bible really says about sex.

You may want to start with Proverbs 5:18–19, a passage too few husbands know:

> May your fountain be blessed,
>> and may you rejoice in the wife of your youth.
> A loving doe, a graceful deer—
>> may her breasts satisfy you always,
>> may you ever be intoxicated with her love.

"Always" and "ever" mean that sexual intimacy should be a thriving part of your marriage for its entire length, starting today.

15. Childhood Abuse

Tara's husband grew up being abused—verbally, emotionally, and sexually—by more than one perpetrator. While she knew something of his abuse before they married, she didn't have the full story and certainly didn't realize how it would impact their sex life. She found herself as a wife not understanding why he resisted sex or seemed so disengaged when they did have it.

> He was trying to protect me in his mind. He's going, *Sexual abuse is ugly and awful. I don't want you to have to deal with sexual abuse because it's icky and awful, so I'm going to protect you from it.* So what he did was protect me from it six feet away. . . . But then we had six-foot distance because he didn't want me to hurt.

Jesus Loves Children

When people brought children to Jesus to receive a blessing, his close disciples saw this as an imposition on the Messiah's limited time and wanted them to stop. Jesus answered, "Let the children come to me, and do not hinder them, for to such belongs the kingdom of God" (Luke 18:16 ESV). Perhaps it was a child's innocence, curiosity, willingness to believe, and reliance on a parent that Jesus was thinking about.

But of course, our Lord knows that too many children don't remain innocent and can't rely on their earthly parent, even if their heavenly parent is trustworthy. Too many children are victims of child abuse or neglect.

Was your husband one of them?

Maltreatment Is Common

About one in seven children in the US has experienced child abuse and/or neglect in the last year.[1] Imagine how many adults are walking around with child abuse in their background. It's both shocking and heartbreaking.

The most common maltreatment is neglect, followed by physical abuse, sexual abuse, and psychological abuse. But however maltreatment manifests, a child's woundedness can show up in various ways later in life, including the area of sexuality. It can impact how they view themselves, how they interpret others' actions, what they believe about sex, and much more.

While many adults who endured child abuse recognize they were mistreated, plenty do not. They don't recognize what they experienced as abuse, perhaps believing their parents were simply strict or they were a "bad kid" who deserved some of what happened to them.

Either way, many men don't want to talk about it. It's natural for those abused to avoid the topic and the pain it can stir up, but men in particular have been socialized to avoid admitting they were victims, to downplay emotional pain, and to "man up" and "get over it." They may have difficulty coming up with words to describe what happened to them or how it made them feel.

Yet they live every day with the consequences. And if it's impacted your marriage's intimacy, you do too.

Your Body Knows

In 2015, Bessel van der Kolk summarized his life's work in *The Body Keeps the Score*. Having worked with trauma victims—from tough combat veterans to fragile, abused children—he noted,

Trauma, by definition, is unbearable and intolerable. Most rape victims, combat soldiers, and children who have been molested become so upset when they think about what they experienced that they try to push it out of their minds, try to act as if nothing happened, and move on. It takes tremendous energy to keep functioning while carrying the memory of terror and the shame of utter weakness and vulnerability. While we all want to move beyond trauma, the part of our brain that is devoted to ensuring our survival, deep below our rational brain, is not very good at denial.[2]

In the face of a terrible threat, our prefrontal cortex—the "rational brain"—goes offline, and the emotional brain and "reptilian brain," known for survival instinct, kick in. Everything inside us simply screams "NO!" and we're viscerally motivated to move to safety.

But sometimes we can't. A child cannot stop abuse or neglect. And that trauma becomes seared inside them. As the title of Dr. van der Kolk's book says, the body keeps the score. "Trauma produces actual physiological changes, including a recalibration of the brain's alarm system, an increase in stress hormone activity, and alterations in the system that filters relevant information from irrelevant."[3]

If your husband experienced abuse, his physiology was affected at such a deep level that he likely can't even explain why he's shutting down. That would require the rational brain's involvement, but the problem lies so much deeper.

He may simply have a visceral resistance to sexual intimacy, or other intimacy, in your marriage. Getting close can retrigger the trauma.

A Safe Place

But you're safe, right? That's what you want your husband to know—that whatever happened to him before, you're a safe place to land, a person who'll treat him with kindness and goodness, the one he can trust. If he could believe that, surely his desire would return and your sexual relationship would be fine.

Except it doesn't work that way. His automatic reactions are embedded in the nervous system, and *knowing* he's safe isn't the same as *feeling* he's safe. The prefrontal cortex can't just tell the reptilian brain to calm down. That mental lizard screams "NO!" when it senses physical or emotional survival is at risk.

Let's say you cozy up to your husband on the couch, wrap your arms around him, and say, "I want you, now." Many men would see that as a sexy invitation, but a victim of physical or sexual childhood abuse might feel trapped between the couch arm and your body, the wrap of your arms subconsciously reminding him of when he was held in place, and your assertive statement feeling like an aggressor's demand. Without thinking, his body reacts. His breath catches, his muscles tighten, his rational brain goes offline, and something inside him yells, *No, not again.*

A triggered husband may become visibly agitated or distant or simply find a way to extricate himself from the situation. And he may not know why he isn't interested in what you're offering. He just feels he has to protect himself as best he can.

As Dr. van der Kolk explains,

> Achieving any sort of deep intimacy—a close embrace, sleeping with a mate, and sex—requires allowing oneself to experience immobilization without fear. It is especially challenging for traumatized people to discern when they are actually safe and to be able to activate their defenses when they are in danger. This requires having experiences that can restore the sense of physical safety.[4]

What experiences can restore that sense of safety? What can convince your husband that you're a safe place for sexual intimacy when his internal system automatically raises barriers to avoid closeness, vulnerability, and authenticity?

Tara found that her husband needed time to purge bad memories of the abuse and his victimizers that popped into his mind at times:

> Another revelation was when he said, "Honey, there are other people in our bed." I realized that was why he was distracted.
>
> He was able to tell me what he needed: "When we first get started, all those things are in my head. It takes a few minutes to clear them out." I took his words to heart. He needs a few minutes to clear his head. So instead of me being mad at him, I'm just going to allow that it might take him a few minutes to clear it out. And that was because he did want to be with me, and only me. That was a good thing.

Tara and her husband worked hard to restore a sense of safety for him, including giving him time to mentally prepare and allowing him an escape hatch. "I would sometimes hold him and simply say, 'Babe, this time's not gonna work. It's okay.' And he almost always had to hear that. Like, *I have an out.*"

Knowing that he could say no without repercussions helped him over time to feel safe and say yes.

Same Trauma, Different Response

If your husband has shared stories of childhood abuse with you, or if you suspect he went through trauma, please, please do not rely on what I say here. Find a trauma-informed counselor or coach who can walk you both through restoring that sense of safety. And if you've experienced trauma, you likely need to seek help for yourself first. Even if you think you're over it, your body may have held on to those memories in secret places you haven't yet realized. You should work through your own issues and get to a healthy place that's good for your own well-being, your husband's healing, and the strength of your marriage.

But I'll summarize what experts advise to let you know what direction you may need to head.

First, talking it out isn't enough. Some people think that once the abuse stories are out there, the work is done. But while acknowledging what happened is a necessary step, it's insufficient to resolve the issues. As we've noted, the body kept score and will continue to react when it senses danger, even when the rational brain knows *that was then, this is now.*

Second, if the problem involves the body, the solution also involves the body. That is, whatever the form of abuse, the body reacts to and remembers what happened. Treating trauma effectively often involves revisiting the trauma and rehearsing different physical reactions to retrain the body and mind. That could involve mindfulness, neurofeedback, eye movement desensitization and reprocessing (EMDR), drama, or something else. But the goal is to help the abuse survivor identify triggers, cope with intense emotions, self-soothe, and exert personal agency. While I encourage your husband to seek out a trauma-informed therapist, if that option is not available, he can read up on how trauma manifests with *The Body Keeps the Score*, seek support groups for abuse survivors, and learn mind and body techniques that can interrupt automatic negative responses to triggers.

Third, intimacy matters. While it may take time for your husband to feel comfortable with sexual intimacy, you can invest in other forms of intimacy that can help him process his past pain and reinvent his perspective today.

While your husband wasn't protected properly as a child, you can reassure him now with your voice, your embrace, your listening ear, your shoulder to cry on, your understanding and patience, your support for him getting the help he needs. You can share how deeply you mourn for the little boy he was, who was mistreated and has carried those wounds for far too long. You can be that "friend who sticks closer than a brother" (Prov. 18:24)—reliable, loving, and providing hope.

Finally, pushing your husband to deal with trauma before he's ready can retraumatize him. Yeah, I know that feels like a no-win situation. If he needs to deal with something to be healthy, then shouldn't you be able to tell him that and even insist on it? While that may seem reasonable to you, trauma experts advise waiting until someone feels truly safe before even asking for their story. Even then, the story may come out in bits and pieces and over the course of days, weeks, months, or even years. You may need to pave the way, indicating your willingness to listen and support him, before he's able to put words to what happened. Go slow, pray for wisdom, and be there consistently and compassionately.

Tara and her husband, Joe, worked through their issues and built a beautiful marriage, so much so that they now host the *Behind Our Smiles* podcast, where they share marriage advice. Tara provided additional insights for wives whose husbands experienced abuse, sexual or otherwise.

First, she noted her husband needed more space. "I couldn't just come up to him and start kissing him. That was not helpful." Rather, she asked if she could touch him and told him why. "I'd say, 'We're having a connection here, and I want to express our connection physically,' versus him just hearing, 'I want something from you.' He needed to know I wasn't trying to take something from him."

Second, she had to be persistent and patient. "I had to keep trying and be patient with the process. If we don't get it right away, it's okay. If he can't be everything I want him to be right now, it's okay."

Third, her husband's body had been so misused, she had to show extra sensitivity. "I had to be gentle with his body. I let him know I love his body, and it's a source of joy for me. It's beautiful and it's not damaged. And it's mine now. Not in a possessive way, but like 'I will caretake for you now. I can be your caretaker even though I know that it hasn't always been cared for.'"

Finally, she reassured him that he'd been treated unfairly and carried no responsibility for what had happened to him. "I had to remind him it wasn't his fault. And it wasn't his fault and it wasn't his fault. I still tell my husband that to this day, and he still appreciates it."

Bit by bit, safe moment by safe moment, Tara helped her husband to feel secure and loved in their bedroom and to know he had full control regarding participation in their sex life. Over time, his present positive experiences with his wife overshadowed the pain of his past.

Overcoming trauma can feel like a too-heavy undertaking for both the victim and their spouse, but Tara and others have found answers, healing, and satisfying sexual intimacy. And so can you.

MENTAL AND EMOTIONAL FACTORS

The phrase "my heart" appears in the Psalms 55 times, as psalmists share their feelings and cry out to God for his intervention. That's about every 545 words that "my heart" is mentioned in this book that is filled with emotion.

In Song of Songs, a book of love poetry between a husband and wife, "my heart" shows up only 8 times. But that's about every 250 words, making its appearance even more frequent.

In both of these wisdom books, one thing is clear: our hearts matter deeply to God and to the sexual relationship we have with our covenant mate.

Unfortunately, many of us have wounded hearts or psyches that make engaging in lovemaking more difficult than it should be. Let's talk about what we can do about them.

16. Body Image

For approximately forever, women have been judged on their external beauty. The pressure to be physically attractive comes at us from all angles—from society to media to community to family. Indeed, marketers try particularly hard to convince us that we're not pretty enough without X product or service, and the number of messages that come at us can feel like a barrage of missiles.

Having heard from so many wives about how body image issues disturb their ability to engage sexually, I've often written on this topic and invited guests to post about it on my site, hoping to help women feel that yes, they are enough, they are beautiful.

But men have body image issues too. Some husbands are so self-conscious about their perceived flaws, they aren't eager to get naked and have sex.

What Makes Someone Attractive?

There was this guy in college—we'll call him Ed. Because his name was Ed. (It's not like he's going to read this book.) One day I was talking with several other girls after Ed had come by the table, chatted with us for a bit, and left. We all agreed that he was really cute and totally dateable.

Was Ed a classic hottie like someone you'd see on a romance novel or a *GQ* cover? No, but he was such a positive, charming, engaging guy that over time, all of us gals concluded he was extremely attractive.

Many individuals miss this aspect of attraction. We act like there's some set standard of hotness we must reach to feel good about ourselves. The truth is that we're attractive because of who we are.

Not to mention that people have types. I'm a fan of tall and lanky, but one of my closest friends likes barrel-chested men with thicker frames. I'm a fan of classic men's hairstyles, while another bestie goes wild for her husband's longer, mussy hair. I like beards, and yet another friend dislikes facial hair.

I suspect the man you chose was handsome to you for various reasons—both external features and personality factors that shone through in his looks. If only your husband could believe that you really love him just the way he is.

Comparison Is the Thief of Joy

Have you heard the saying "Comparison is the thief of joy"?[1] It's a wise observation, yet we compare all the time.

It's instinct for us to look at others and consider how we differ. And it's a short step to then thinking we don't measure up in some way. You do it, I do it, and our husbands do it.

Some husbands do it about their looks. Comparison in this area is different for men in that standards of attractiveness show up in more masculine ways. That unrealistic standard often involves low body fat, well-defined jaws, and more six-packs than your local liquor store.

But just like most women don't look like airbrushed magazine models, most men don't look like personal fitness trainers. And yet, a lot of men think they should look like that. Maybe because they want to feel good about themselves, or maybe because they want their wife to have the very best.

Many Women Aren't Helping

I'm regularly surprised by how many women—Christian women, mind you—are vocal about which celebrities they think are sexy. It could be the latest actor in a superhero movie, a favorite sports player, or some random photo they saw on Instagram.

Some of these same women would cry foul (or "lust!") if a husband ogled and commented on a woman's appearance in the same way. So what are we saying to men by engaging in the same actions women have decried for years—viewing people as a collection of body parts and dwelling on their sex appeal?

No wonder certain men begin to question whether they measure up. When they look in the mirror or down at their midsection, they don't see six-pack abs. They're lucky to have a two-pack, and quite a few are sporting a keg.

If we turn around and reassure our husband that he's our hottie, does he hear that past the static of how we talked about this or that actor, model, or athlete? Let's gain control of our thoughts and our tongues and not make body image a bigger issue for men who are struggling.

A Word About Penis Size

How big is big enough? That's not only a question I've received from men but one that swirls around in the heads of many men. While they may be loud and proud about having a penis, plenty of husbands secretly wonder if their penis is sufficient for their wife.

A 2006 internet survey of 52,031 heterosexual men and women concluded that while only 55% of men were satisfied with their size, 85% of women were content with their partner's size.[2] Also, many men don't recognize the common parameters of penis size—that is, where penile length and girth (the measurement all the way around) would fall on a bell curve.

When it comes to penis size, what is typical? Well, we don't know the exact length and girth of the average penis, because it's hard to measure, or to measure it hard. (Hope you chuckled like I did.) To get a good measurement, you need a representative sample of the male population all measuring their erect penises with the same method—ideally, by a trained researcher. And what representative sample is going to agree to that?!

So our best studies involve men who are instructed how to measure and then to self-report. By that framework, the average length (erect) was estimated to be 5.1–5.6 inches, and girth around 4.6 inches.[3] Most men's penis size falls close to those averages. Of 15,000 men studied, only 5% were at or below 4 inches long or 3.8 inches around.[4] But doctors don't advise treatment for penile length unless it's 3 inches or less, because 3 inches is all you need to get the job done and done well.

Do women want their partner to have an above average penis? Some do.[5] But even then, only slightly above average.[6] Most wives are satisfied with their husband's penis.[7] After all, it's not just the size but the man it belongs to that matters to us!

Still, a husband who doesn't feel good about his penis may be less willing to have sex. He could avoid sex altogether, be reluctant to engage, or not be the one to initiate. Getting naked reveals both the penis he's not happy with and his emotional vulnerability.

A few men avoid sex because they believe their penis is too big for their wife's comfort . . . and some of them are right. But this can be addressed with more lubrication and sexual positioning, and having sex less often is likely to make intercourse more challenging because her body doesn't have the opportunity to stretch and adapt.

So how can you reassure him? The answer may not be what you expect. Much like a few compliments of "you're beautiful" cannot erase a woman's lifetime of societal pressure to be prettier, reassuring a husband that his penis is fine won't wipe away his self-doubt. You may need to share some data with him so he can adjust his expectations of what's normal. You may want to ask about his concerns, listen to why it matters to him, and respond to the feelings rather than the size. For example, "That must have been difficult for you, not feeling like you're enough." You may want to explain what you like about his penis, not only its size but also how it fits into your hand or feels inside you. And you can ask, "What can I do to help you feel good about your penis?" He may have an idea in his mind that he hadn't thought to articulate or didn't feel comfortable discussing until you asked—and it may be something you can easily do.

How a husband feels about his body can have a long-term impact on his willingness to bare and share that body. Let's help him feel good about the body that is "awesomely and wonderfully made" by God (Ps. 139:14 NASB).

17. Fatherhood Fears

You're not the only one worried about getting pregnant. Or maybe you're not worried, yet he is. He could even seem excited about having a(nother) kid while experiencing doubt. Fears of first-time fatherhood or expanding his role can dampen a husband's sexual interest.

Not Ready for Children

The only foolproof birth control is abstinence. Otherwise, if he's making sperm and you're making eggs, there's some chance for conception. Even the pill with its 99% effective rate (used properly) means every 1 out of 100 times, you ain't protected. If you have sex even once a week, you reach that one-hundredth time every couple of years.

For some guys, that's nerve-racking. Their worry could stem from a past scare when you (or a prior lover) seemed to be pregnant and he didn't feel ready, or from ingrained messages about not getting a girl pregnant before you're prepared emotionally, financially, or otherwise. He might not trust that he'll be a good father for that first kid or for more kids than he has now. Whatever the reason, his interest and pleasure in sex are diminished by concern about conceiving children he's not ready for.

How can you address this? Talk to him about your family plans, contraception, and what you'll do if a surprise baby happens. If you really want to put things off, you could use two birth control methods until you're ready.

However, consult with your healthcare provider and research contraception. Hormonal birth control can have problematic outcomes for women, including changes in mood and sexual desire.[1] But there are many birth control options, including barrier methods such as condoms and diaphragms, intrauterine devices, natural family planning, and hormonal contraception for women who don't experience negative side effects. Do your homework and discuss alternatives with your husband.

Everything Will Change

Perhaps your husband looks forward to growing your family! But underneath his excitement lies concern or dread that everything will change once baby arrives.

He recognizes that your relationship will get less time and focus. Your finances may be strained, with diapers and daycare dipping into the bank account. His friendships won't remain strong, as he prioritizes family above guys' nights out or finds less in common with non-fathers. And he just won't have as much freedom.

With all that in mind, he may find himself slow-walking his way to parenthood, starting with slow-walking to the bedroom.

One key to transitioning well is discussing expectations. Share your fears first, and let him follow. Acknowledge that parents have less freedom to do what they want to do, and marriages often experience a decrease in satisfaction when children arrive. But in the long run, parents report an increased sense of purpose and meaning in their lives,[2] and marriages can make it through without huge drops in happiness and recover any losses over time.

Suggest concrete ways you can troubleshoot challenges as they come, such as monthly date nights to stay in touch or one or both of you pursuing a side gig for more income. Discuss the seasons of marriage—not just the negatives but the positives that come with them—so that you can look forward to each new stage.

And you know what? Everything will change, whether you have kids or not. That's life, and it unfolds without us knowing what's in store. If you both want kids, you might as well embrace parenthood as part of that big adventure.

Big Shoes to Fill

Whether it's the first kid or the eighth, some men want to be a good dad so much that they worry about becoming a dad at all or again. Their ideal conception of dad comes with big shoes they don't know if they can fill.

Of course, we ladies feel great responsibility as well, but our concerns tend to be different. While we tend to worry about our ability to nurture our children, to detect their wishes, and to provide for everyday needs, men worry about protecting their children, providing materially for them, and sharing dad-like wisdom. Not to mention the pressure to tell great dad jokes.

If this fear runs deep, it could relate to childhood experiences—from an excellent father he doesn't feel he can live up to, to a terrible father he fears replicating, to something in between. If you haven't talked about your families of origin, this may be the time. If there's trauma in his background, encourage him to seek counseling or a support group to work through his understandable hurt and worry.

If it's more that the task feels daunting, reassure him that he'll be a great father and he won't be parenting alone. Suggest ways you can prepare for parenthood—from babysitting friends' children to taking courses. And later, fully incorporate your husband in baby preparations and care, thus developing his confidence and comfort level.

God's Got This

One primary purpose of sexual intimacy is procreation. It's not the only one, yet it's how we as a people fulfill God's early command to "be fruitful and multiply" (Gen. 1:22 NKJV). But he doesn't leave it there. His Word equips parents to bring up children "in wisdom and stature, and in favor with God and man" (Luke 2:52).

If a child comes from your sexual union, God can help you prepare for, provide for, and nurture that child. Parenthood isn't easy, but it's been done successfully countless times throughout history, and you can do it too. Not perfectly, because perfection is God's territory. We just have to love well.

And fostering intimacy now can pay dividends later, because the best environment for a child is one where husband and wife show affection, flirt, and, yes, have sex behind closed doors.

18. Depression and Anxiety

Has your husband experienced depression or anxiety? It may not be easy to tell, because mood disorders in men can look different from those in women. They could come across as apathy or anger, an unusually (for him) short fuse, or just shutting down.

Let's talk about these challenges and whether they might be affecting your husband's willingness to woo.

Too Down to Go Downtown

Everyone from Billie Holiday to Johnny Cash to The Doors has sung about having the blues. James Taylor even titled one song "Everybody Has the Blues." And it's true—everyone feels down from time to time.

But depression is not just having the blues. It's not merely feelings of sadness or irritability but rather a physiological state that results in feelings of sadness or irritability. Depression alters the chemistry in a person's brain, which then sends signals to their body to check out in different ways.

One tool commonly used to diagnose depression is the PHQ-9 (Patient Health Questionnaire-9), and its nine questions inquire about:

- inability to experience pleasure (anhedonia)
- feelings of sadness or hopelessness

- sleep disturbances
- fatigue
- changes in appetite
- feeling bad about yourself
- difficulty concentrating
- obviously slower movement or fidgety behavior
- suicidal thoughts[1]

While this assessment has helped clinicians to identify many folks with depression, it's missed some men because of its focus on feelings, which many men struggle to recognize, and its omission of symptoms that men are more likely to experience. The Mayo Clinic suggests additional signs of male depression:

- escapist behavior, such as spending a lot of time at work or on sports
- physical symptoms, such as headaches, digestive problems, and pain
- problems with alcohol or drug use
- controlling, violent, or abusive behavior
- irritability or inappropriate anger
- risky behavior, such as reckless driving[2]

Do any of those sound familiar?

Now, before you diagnose your husband with depression and insist he get treatment, recognize that all of these criteria can be symptoms of other issues. For instance, not every controlling or violent husband is depressed, and having raised two sons, I can say that risky behavior is fairly typical for young men.

We're simply looking at this issue because it might be part of the challenge with sexual intimacy in your marriage. But depression isn't the only mood disorder that could affect your husband's sexual desire.

Too Distressed to Get Undressed

Singer Bobby McFerrin prescribed, "Don't Worry, Be Happy"—a song about as opposite the blues as one can get. It's a nice sentiment to find reasons for joy even in the worst of circumstances, but it's entirely unrealistic for someone with an anxiety disorder. They can't just stop worrying and be happier, and persistently telling them to do so is likely to add to their anxiety, not decrease it.

What's an anxiety disorder? That term covers phobias, social anxiety, panic disorder, generalized anxiety disorder (GAD), and more. Covering each of these is a task beyond the scope of this book, so let's look at anxiety on the whole.

While we all get anxious from time to time, an anxiety disorder involves persistent, excessive feelings of worry or dread that interfere with everyday functioning. The diagnostic criteria for GAD include:

- feeling restless, keyed up, or on edge
- being easily fatigued
- difficulty concentrating or mind going blank
- irritability
- muscle tension
- sleep disturbance (difficulty falling or staying asleep, or restless, unsatisfying sleep)[3]

Notice a big overlap with depression? That's because they're both mood disorders and can disrupt our lives in similar ways. I have an interesting comparison in my own family: I've suffered from depression, while a relative of mine has dealt with an anxiety disorder. (Both of us received treatment and feel much better now.) While my mood disorder shut me down, her mood disorder stirred her up. She described her experience this way: "Clenched muscles, a thumping heart, sweaty palms, hypervigilance, sensitivity

114

to sudden movements and loud sounds, and constant low-grade fear. It's exhausting." Of course, these are only two examples, and depression and anxiety manifest differently from person to person.

Only recently have experts begun to study how anxiety disorders manifest differently in men than women. Researchers have noted that men are more likely to turn to alcohol and drugs, to attempt release of tension through physical activity, and to express anxiety as anger.[4] In addition, a man's fear is often followed by shame.

When I asked male Facebook followers to share phrases men use with each other to let them know it's not cool to express fear, they delivered quite a list. Imagine for a moment being a guy and having these phrases tossed at you all your life:

"What a wuss."

"Toughen up, princess."

"Turn in your man card."

"Take a spoon of cement and harden up."

"Grow a pair."

So while women may express their worries and fears, men's anxiety often comes out in male-accepted ways, such as social distancing, physical ailments, alcohol or drug use (to calm rampant thoughts), irritability, and frustrated rants. A woman with an anxiety disorder likely feels freer to share her worries and cry, but a man with the same issues struggles to put into words why he's on edge all the time. It's also difficult to express that his anxious thoughts crowd out sexual interest. In fact, his anxiety may involve the bedroom— including worry or fear about his body, his performance, his lack of sex drive, and more. To really enjoy sex, you have to be able to let go a little, and an anxiety disorder won't let go.

Again, just because your husband exhibits some of these symptoms doesn't mean he has an anxiety disorder. But he might, so we're adding it to our "could be" list.

How Can You Help?

What if depression or anxiety *is* impairing your husband's sexual interest or is a contributing factor? What next?

First, talk about depression or anxiety with your husband. Some men don't want to admit they're struggling because depression and anxiety have been associated more with feelings and women. Moreover, the Christian community has sometimes addressed mood disorders as weakness or a lack of faith. But as I said, this isn't selfishly dwelling on our feelings but rather a physiological issue that impacts our emotions. You may want to avoid labels for now, since they can be off-putting for many at first, but clarify that what you're concerned about with him is no less real than high blood pressure or a torn ligament.

Second, encourage your husband to see a clinician and get a proper diagnosis. Any physician can use a diagnostic tool like the PHQ-9, but mental health professionals have more training in identifying and treating mood disorders and differentiating whether they're depression, anxiety, or something else. A psychiatrist can also prescribe and monitor medications if needed. Check your insurance and local resources to see what's available to him.

Third, discuss treatment options. His doctor may suggest antidepressants or talk therapy. Both have good outcomes, but if they make your husband uncomfortable, talk about alternatives or additions. Regular exercise, sunlight, and massage have also helped those with mild-to-moderate mood disorders. And certain dietary supplements, as directed by a healthcare provider or dietitian, could help your particular guy.

Fourth, support his treatment. If exercise helps his brain chemistry get back on track, offer to take that walk with him, go to the gym, sign up for coed softball, etc. If he has to start new medication, encourage him to set reminders to take it. If regular massages are helpful, gift him with one or sign up for a couples' massage. Do what you can to be his cheerleader as he fights back against depression or anxiety.

Fifth, help him monitor the impact. Is he improving? Do you feel like you're seeing more of the guy you once knew? Does he report feeling better? If one treatment isn't having a strong enough impact, that doesn't mean he should stop all treatment. With medication, for example, it can take time to find the right one at the right dosage. And how's your sex life? Some medications can ease depression or anxiety but dampen sexual interest, while others won't have that effect for him. Anticipate adjustments to the plan as you move forward.

Finally, keep talking. Don't nag him, but keep the lines of communication open and positive. Your husband will probably need reassurance from time to time. Remember how one symptom of depression is feeling bad about yourself? Being diagnosed with depression or anxiety comes across to some as one more reason to feel bad about themselves. *Why is everyone else okay but I'm not coping? Will I always have to take medication to feel normal? What will my friends or family think?*

You can be your husband's touch point by reminding him that life struggles are normal, that treatments are not altering him but getting the real him back, and that he's got an ally in his corner. Don't aim for platitudes—which never work with depression or anxiety anyway—but validate his concerns while sharing your confidence that things can and will get better.

What About Faith?

It doesn't help a person with a mood disorder when someone cites Scriptures like, "Be of good cheer" (John 16:33 NKJV) or "Do not worry" (Matt. 6:25). Well-meaning believers who share these in an effort to encourage don't fully understand what major depression or an anxiety disorder is. They think of them as fleeting feelings of sadness or worry, when they're a full-body experience that cannot be wished or prayed away.

That does not mean God has no role in all of this. Of course he does! Scripture says that he is with those who are brokenhearted and anxious. Time spent with him can ease our burden and buoy our spirits.

Consider what Paul said in 2 Corinthians 7:6: "But God, who comforts the downcast, comforted us by the coming of Titus." God's spiritual comfort came in the tangible form of Titus, who likely brought provisions as well as encouragement and companionship. In the same way, God helping us through depression or anxiety can come through both his presence and what he provides through others. Reaching out for therapy or medication doesn't mean you're shortchanging your faith. Accept the whole healing that God brings.

19. Stress

I wavered on whether to put this chapter under "Physical Health" or "Mental and Emotional Factors," because stress straddles those two categories like a fence-sitting cowboy. Regardless, when it comes to husbands whose sex drive has dropped, stress is one of the core reasons. Other factors can complicate the issue, but the pressure of work, finances, fatherhood, and other day-to-day challenges accounts for a fair amount of sexual disinterest.

Under Pressure

Stress affects us all, but some seasons are worse than others and some people handle it better than others.

When an HDW tells me her husband isn't interested, I often ask what he does for a living. If he's holding down more than one job, overseeing a time-sensitive project at work, or running a family farm on his own, we might have found the answer for his lack of desire. He's feeling pressure to perform and provide, two objectives most men prioritize. Most husbands want to do a job well and bring in enough income to care for their family. Laudable goals, but all that pressure can affect his sexual interest, as well as his ability to perform in the bedroom.

Tiffany remembers a particularly difficult season. "The job was very stressful. . . . I was getting half my husband when he came home. He wanted to sit in his nothing box. He wanted to watch TV. He wanted to just not engage, so I had to work really hard at getting his attention."

Yet it may not be the amount of work required but rather how he feels about what he's doing.

Megan notices improvement when her husband's military service is going well. "There will be seasons where sex gets better, and I see that it's tied to if he's really happy with his job, if he's feeling pumped up. When he decided to go active duty and he was away at training, he was close enough that I could go visit him. I would get long weekends from work, and it was like, 'This is the most romantic, amazing time.' We're in this hotel room, and we would have sex, and he would be not scared, not nervous. He was happy with it, but he was also very happy with how he was doing in training."

Megan's story illustrates how a couple's sex life can benefit when things are going well. But how can you manage those times when stress hinders his availability and interest?

If it's just a season, you may need to set the bar lower on frequency, come up with options to maintain some sexual intimacy, and hang in there, being patient and waiting until the major stress passes. That could include scheduling sex with your husband at a time he might be more available, asking for him to clear his schedule now and then, or getting creative about what time of day to make love. For instance, some men do better with morning sex, when the stress of the day hasn't kicked in yet.

If stress is a way of life, however, you may want to discuss what changes need to happen. Many men overestimate how much income their wives expect them to bring in and underestimate how much she'd rather have his presence than a bigger paycheck. It may take a few conversations to convince him that you're willing to cut back or find other ways to bring in income so he can be home and relaxed more often. You may have to increase stress for the short term, such as adding schooling or training for one or both of you, to get to a better place in the future. But if stress is ongoing and you can't see an end in sight, the lack of sex isn't your main problem anyway—you need more time together as a couple for the health of your marriage.

Or maybe circumstances aren't that bad, but your husband simply experiences stress more intensely. We all know folks who are almost too relaxed about life, with nothing seeming to make a ripple in the calm of their demeanor. And we know folks who absorb stress like a thirsty sponge. Did you marry one?

If so, start with compassion. I once knew a woman who wore stress like a fashion trend she'd never give up, and many found her difficult to be around. But when I imagined what it would be like to wake up every day and be her, it changed the way I engaged with her. She really and truly did not know how to let go.

Now, of course, such people would do well to get help and find ways to de-stress! That's why I said "start with compassion," not end there. When you recognize how painful it must be to carry such a burden, then you can better come alongside your husband and advocate for him to find healthier ways of coping with the stress of life.

Acknowledge his personality and challenges, but also lovingly let him know he cannot continue to live at that level of stress without damage to his health, his well-being, and his relationships, including the sexual one with you.

Stress Saps the Body

Speaking of health, stress changes our physiology. Whenever we're stressed, our bodies respond by releasing hormones that refocus our attention on the problem at hand. Heart rate increases, breathing quickens, muscles tighten, and blood pressure rises, all so that we can react to the stressor.[1] After the crisis passes, our bodies release other hormones that settle us back down.

But chronic stress keeps our bodies at that heightened level and overtaxes our system, resulting in long-term issues such as:

- headaches
- digestive problems
- body aches and pains
- insomnia
- frequent colds and infections
- loss of sexual desire and/or ability
- obesity
- cardiovascular disease[2]

Regarding sexuality specifically, high stress shuts down reproductive activity in the body for a time so that having sex becomes less important when a person is facing a life-threatening situation. Or it should. Chronic stress impacts our reproductive systems even more—lowering testosterone for men, making erection more difficult, and decreasing fertility.

The main stress hormone, cortisol, is effective as a fight-or-flight signal, but it's also a libido killer. Over time, it makes the whole body feel bad and saps one's willingness and capacity to have sex.

Too Knackered for Nooky

I love Britishisms, including Cockney slang and words like "chuffed," "nutter," and especially "knackered," which means worn out. But not just worn out—more like bone-tired or fully drained.

Overstressed men can also find themselves too knackered for nooky. They may experience mental fatigue from work and worry; emotional fatigue from dealing with people at work, caring for kids, or managing their own feelings; or physical fatigue from work and physiological changes. This exhaustion isn't due to a lack of sleep per se but rather stress siphoning their reserves.

122

You may look at the situation and think that you wouldn't be knackered from all that he does. Hey, maybe you're doing more than him! But how much stress exhausts someone depends a lot on their personality. I can easily put in long days . . . unless it involves crowds, in which case this introvert will return home feeling like a popped balloon. My extrovert friends don't feel the same, because all that people interaction doesn't stress them out like it does me. When thinking about what's stressful for your mate, consider who they are, not how you would see the situation.

How to Shoo Away Stress

Numerous sources note that sex, especially when it ends with orgasm, relieves stress and activates the release of relaxing hormones, such as endorphins, oxytocin, and prolactin. Plus, sex causes the stress hormone, cortisol, to decrease, along with blood pressure.[3]

While those are all positive perks that can lower stress, there's a catch. One must be able to relax enough to enjoy sex for that release of tension to happen. And sadly, stress makes it difficult to have the physical energy, the mental focus, and the sexual desire or responsiveness to sexual stimuli that are needed to enjoy sex.

My marriage experienced a dry spell when my husband was working a job he didn't like that much, couldn't get sufficient staff to cover all the bases, and put in so much overtime that we rarely got to eat dinner together. He'd been busy before, so I didn't make the connection until we went on a cruise where no one from work could reach him. Suddenly, his sex drive was back! I realized it wasn't me; it was the two-ton weight of stress on his shoulders that had been lifted during our weeklong vacation. When we got back, his sexual interest dropped a bit (hey, we weren't on vacation anymore!), but not back to the low it had been before, because we knew the reason and could work on reducing his stress.

How can you reduce stress? Experts say it mostly comes down to three areas.[4]

Be Social. Having family and friends with whom we regularly engage lowers our stress levels and increases our lifespan. Unfortunately, many men find it difficult to make friends. According to a 2021 American Perspectives Survey,

> Thirty years ago, a majority of men (55 percent) reported having at least six close friends. Today, that number has been cut in half. Slightly more than one in four (27 percent) men have six or more close friends today. Fifteen percent of men have no close friendships at all, a fivefold increase since 1990.[5]

How can you help your husband reach out? You can encourage him to reconnect with someone he was once close to or have a guys' night out or in, suggest a double date with a couple you both enjoy, or sign you both up for a social activity with your church. Don't just schedule an adult version of a playdate for him, but rather seek his input and make it clear you want him to have companions who can help him relax and refocus on the good things in life. You can also find ways to be social with one another, like going out to dinner or even the grocery store together and setting a boundary of no talking about work, kids, politics, or anything else that makes him tense during a date.

Connecting with others and with you could relieve some of the stress that gets in the way of his sexual desire and satisfaction.

Be Physical. Not in the "let's get physical" sense that Olivia Newton-John sang about—though we're not opposed to that here!—but rather moving the body. Exercise requires deep breathing and loosens the muscles, both of which can reduce your husband's stress. It can be anything from an intensive, competitive sport to a brisk walk to slower movements like tai chi.

If he's not eager to exercise himself, do it together. Even a walk around the neighborhood can reset stress levels. Or try dancing in the living room, letting both the physical activity and the oxytocin of a long embrace ease tension. That might set the mood then or later for that other physical stuff.

Be Calm. Scripture has a lot to say about the importance of rest. God gave us one day a week to rest, as he did after creating the world, and his Son said, "Come to me, all you who are weary and burdened, and I will give you rest" (Matt. 11:28). God wants us to find peace in turmoil, serenity in restlessness.

Calming one's spirit can also reduce the effects of stress, though sometimes that's easier said than done. Your husband can't just will himself to be calm and—ta-da!—peace arrives. But he can take actions to reach a more tranquil state. Among those are meditation and mindfulness. Research bears out the usefulness of these tactics for handling stress. But too often, they get a bad rap as being Eastern religious practices. While you can find plenty of meditation resources that focus on the inner self or the "world soul," meditation was also practiced in our faith tradition, way back to Isaac (Gen. 24:63), Joshua (Josh. 1:8), and the psalmists:

> They speak of the glorious splendor of your majesty—
> and I will meditate on your wonderful works. (Ps. 145:5)

> I meditate on your precepts
> and consider your ways. (Ps. 119:15)

Even when things got really stressful, one answer was to meditate:

> Though rulers sit together and slander me,
> your servant will meditate on your decrees. (Ps. 119:23)

You might suggest a time of meditation for you both or that he try it for himself. Many apps can walk you through how meditation works, specifically mental focus and breathing techniques, without following a particular religious practice. But if you come upon an Eastern religion–sounding meditation, you can adapt according to your faith.

I've done both meditation and yoga. When an instructor suggests a mantra or message to guide the day's focus, I pick a Bible verse or phrase. It could be something as simple as "The LORD is my refuge" (Ps. 91:9) or as involved as "Do not be anxious about anything, but in every situation, by prayer and petition, with thanksgiving, present your requests to God" (Phil. 4:6). Those go along with meditation and mindfulness techniques such as paying attention to breathing, letting intrusive thoughts pass through rather than dwelling on or trying to repel them, and focusing on the five senses. All together, they help me to release tension and reclaim God's rest.

Stress can suppress sexual interest, but you can help your husband rediscover rest, peace, and the excitement of sexual intimacy. Encourage him to take that burden to Christ, and offer to carry it with him as well. As Galatians 6:2 says, "Carry each other's burdens, and in this way you will fulfill the law of Christ."

20. Psychiatric Disorders

While the impact of depression and anxiety on sexual functioning has been widely studied by medical and psychological experts, other mental health issues have not received the same attention. There isn't nearly as much research available for issues like post-traumatic stress disorder (PTSD), schizophrenia, and bipolar disorder, but it stands to reason that they would have repercussions for libido and sexual interest. If your husband has been diagnosed with one of these disorders or you believe he might have one of them, you're probably wondering how that plays into the issue you're facing. So let's look into psychiatric disorders and their potential impact.

Psychosis

Psychotic disorders are characterized by abnormal perception and mental processing such as delusions, hallucinations, and disordered thinking. The psychotic disorder that most have heard about is schizophrenia, although there are many misconceptions about it—for instance, believing those with schizophrenia are necessarily violent or that they have multiple personalities.[1] But the main feature of any psychosis is losing touch with reality.[2] That is, those with psychosis have trouble distinguishing what's real and what's not.

In one systematic review of 770 cases, the prevalence of sexual dysfunction while experiencing psychosis spanned from 16.8% to 70%, and in the ultrahigh state—a time of heightened psychosis—it was 50%.[3] But also problematic is how antipsychotic medications can have a dampening effect on sex drive and arousal.

At least half of people who take antipsychotic medication report sexual dysfunction. Most antipsychotic medications block dopamine receptors which can lead to increased serum prolactin levels and reduced sexual arousal (erectile dysfunction in men and reduced vaginal lubrication in women) and libido. Antipsychotic drugs can also impair sexual functioning through sedation and by direct effects on blood flow to reproductive organs.[4]

That feels like a no-win situation, right? But oftentimes adjustments can be made to treatments to alleviate side effects. It's just that the doctor doesn't know unless the patients share their experience. While physicians should screen for sexual dysfunction, they may not. In which case it's up to your husband to ask questions, advocate for both his mental and his sexual health, and do what he can to manage both.

PTSD

For far too long, both experts and individuals didn't appreciate how much past trauma plays into sexual problems. Not everyone gets it yet, but many more Christians now recognize that traumatic events can leave a mark on our bodies, minds, and hearts that make genuine intimacy with another beyond difficult.

Mayo Clinic defines PTSD this way:

Post-traumatic stress disorder (PTSD) is a mental health condition that's triggered by a terrifying event—either experiencing it or witnessing it. Symptoms may include flashbacks, nightmares and severe anxiety, as well as uncontrollable thoughts about the event.[5]

Notice that the event could have been experienced—such as being abused as a child (see chapter 15), victimized by violence, or involved in a severe accident—or witnessed, such as seeing someone else abused, wounded, or killed. Moreover, we all experience trauma in life at some point, and just because one person recovers without experiencing PTSD doesn't mean another will. It's not about personal strength or mental fitness but rather how some brains get stuck and need more help to get out of the trauma loop.

While some get diagnosed with PTSD, others don't realize that's what's happening. They feel stuck but don't know why, or they don't understand why their efforts to move on have failed time and time again. But as discussed before, while the consequences of trauma invade at the level of awareness, the trauma itself happens in the body and the brain at an unconscious level. If PTSD is a possibility for your husband, you might want to talk about the definition and the reasons why overcoming without outside assistance is difficult, then seek a healthcare provider to screen for this diagnosis.

PTSD is associated with an increased risk of sexual difficulties, particularly overall sexual function, sexual desire, sexual satisfaction, and sexual distress. Those with PTSD tend to be avoidant and feel bad about themselves, and they may feel numb—in general and regarding sex.[6] If the trauma involved sexual abuse or assault, then problems with desire, arousal, and satisfaction may be even more pronounced.

Sexual abuse is more widespread than many people realize. Prevent Child Abuse America estimates that one in six boys is sexually abused before age 16. Moreover,

> Boys are less likely than girls to report sexual abuse because of fear, the social stigma against homosexual behavior, the desire to appear self-reliant (boys grow up believing that they should not allow themselves to be harmed or talk about painful experiences), and the concern for loss of independence. Furthermore, evidence

suggests that one in every three incidents of child sexual abuse are not remembered by the adults who experienced them, and that the younger the child was at the time of the abuse, and the closer the relationship to the abuser, the more likely one is that the child will not be able to recall the event.[7]

If your husband has been through trauma or if he exhibits some of the symptoms of PTSD, encourage him to seek help. It's a brave thing to reach out and get the assistance needed to heal from trauma.

Bipolar Disorder

Bipolar disorder is aptly named, as those with this brain disorder swing from one extreme emotional state to another during distinct periods of days or weeks. These episodes are either manic/hypomanic (abnormally happy or irritable mood) or depressive (sad mood), though of course there are periods of neutral moods too.

The most common sexual consequences are becoming hypersexual during manic phases and disinterested during depressive phases.[8] This back-and-forth can prove confusing and exhausting to a spouse.

The disinterested times will mirror what was discussed in chapter 18 regarding depression, while overly interested times, in the manic phase, can involve obsessive thinking about sex, a willingness to take risks, and impulsive sexual behaviors. Clearly, neither extreme is good for long-term marital intimacy.

If you've been through such mood swings with your husband, you may want to show him information about bipolar disorder and ask him to visit a healthcare provider to be screened. Treatments include medication but also lifestyle changes that can help him avoid the triggers that send him into a manic or depressive episode. And if your husband has been diagnosed with bipolar disorder but isn't participating in treatment currently, talk with him about your concerns for his overall health and how this disorder has negatively affected your sex life.

Some medications can also impact sex drive, so encourage him to discuss any problems with his doctor and adjust as needed. Even if your husband's overall drive ends up a little lower on average while he's on medication, having more balance means that his sexual interest will reflect his genuine self rather than the mood state he's in. All in all, that's a much better way to build intimacy in the marriage bed.

Other Disorders

When I completed my master's degree in counseling, the mental health community was using the Diagnostic and Statistical Manual (DSM) IV—the authoritative guide for clinicians to diagnose mental disorders. That heavy, cracked-spine book still sits on my shelf. But a lot has happened since 1999, including a new DSM-5. It's so different that they went from Roman numerals to Arabic ones. [grin]

Truth is, whether it's my old DSM-IV or the current DSM-5, the psychiatric manual covers numerous disorders, and if your husband has one of them, it could impair his sexual interest or functioning. If you sense that mental or emotional problems are wreaking havoc not only on his sex life but on his life overall, encourage him to seek help.

Let him know that any diagnosis or treatment he goes through won't lower him in your eyes, but instead you'll see him as heroic for speaking up, getting support, and doing the hard work of healing.

21. Sexual Orientation and Identity

We've all heard the stories—someone marries a person of the opposite sex, then later comes out as gay or lesbian. Perhaps you know someone it happened to. I'm personally familiar with two examples.

If your husband is reluctant to have sex, you may have wondered if he's attracted to men instead of women. Could that be it? Could he be same-sex attracted?[1]

How Prevalent Is Homosexuality?

How likely it is that your husband is a closet gay man depends somewhat on how prevalent homosexuality is in society as a whole. That is, statistically speaking, if a fair number of men turn out to be gay, it's more likely one's own sexually disinterested husband could be among them.

Most people are terrible at guessing the percentage of non-heterosexuals in the general population. A January 2022 YouGov poll showed that respondents wildly overestimated the percentage of Americans who are gay or lesbian (24% versus the actual 3%), bisexual (24% versus 4%), and transgender (12% versus 1%).[2] But hey, they also said that 22% of Americans live in the Lone Star State, and as a born-and-bred Texan myself, I can confirm that we are big but not that big.[3]

Some might argue that the actual percentage of non-heterosexuals isn't higher because people don't want to admit to pollsters that they are gay. However, Gallup has seen this trend for several years in their surveys. In 2002, people guessed 21–22% of Americans were gay, lesbian, or bisexual. In 2012, it was 24.6%, and in 2019, it was 23.6% of the population. In that same time, the percentage of people that researchers estimate to be LGBT doubled . . . from 2% to 4.5%.[4]

That's still not a lot. And plenty of gay and lesbian people are in same-sex relationships already, so how many people married to someone of the opposite sex are likely to be gay or lesbian? We don't know, but probably not many. Even some of those people identify not as exclusively gay or lesbian but as bisexual, meaning that a lack of sexual interest for their opposite-sex spouse isn't because they aren't sexually attracted.

Consequently, I'd rate this reason for a low drive husband as unlikely for most wives reading this book.

But What About Your Husband?

It hardly matters what the general statistics are if you're the one married to—and trying to have sex with—a man who'd rather be with a man. So how can you know if this might be the underlying cause of his disinterest?

The obvious answer is to ask him. But a man may not be ready to admit same-sex attraction, especially to his wife. Moreover, if he's not same-sex attracted, the accusation could feel offensive to him. You may prefer a list of what to look for.

But there's no comprehensive "gaydar" list. The way to know if someone is sexually attracted to the same sex is if they admit or display attraction to the same sex. Here are a few questions to consider:

- Has your husband's lack of sexual interest developed more recently, or has his interest always been low?

- Has your husband shown interest in females in other contexts (for example, having previous girlfriends or noticing pretty women), or has he rarely, if ever, seemed curious about other women?
- Does your husband seem to easily identify with heterosexual men, or does he have a less clear sense of belonging?
- Does your husband have interests more in line with heterosexual men, or do they align more with heterosexual women? (Mind you, plenty of female-focused men love to cook, knit, shop, etc. This is just one question among many.)
- Have all of your husband's romantic experiences involved a woman, or has he ever shared about a prior experience with or attraction to a man?
- Do you have a sense of romance and affection with your husband, or does your whole relationship feel off, as if your husband wants you more as a friend than a lover and life partner?

If you answered yes to the latter half of most or all of these questions, that may, along with other indicators, point to same-sex attraction or confusion. That word "may" matters a lot! These questions are not scientific or definitive. They're only to help you think through the possibilities and begin mulling over the need for evidence to determine what's going on.

A lack of sexual interest alone proves nothing about your husband's sexual orientation. You'd need to see other red flags to recognize sexual orientation as the problem.

Please Don't Assume

There's a famous episode of *Seinfeld* called "The Outing," in which Jerry Seinfeld and his friend George Constanza are mistakenly

labeled as being in a romantic relationship. For the majority of
the episode, they try desperately to correct the record ("We're
not gay!"), all while adding, "Not that there's anything wrong
with that."[5]

Perhaps the reason the show strikes a nerve is because people
do get misidentified as same-sex attracted when they're not. Unfortunately, that can happen to a man who doesn't show the level
of sexual interest in women, particularly his wife, that other guys
consider normal. I've even had readers, typically higher desire
husbands, suggest that any guy who doesn't want sex more than
his wife must be gay. And some women out there might agree.

These erroneous assumptions only add to the problem. After
all, why would a heterosexual man want to admit his lower desire
and even get help if doing so will put him in the situation Jerry and
George found themselves? Not wanting to be accused of same-sex
attraction, he may avoid sex, or even the topic of sex, even more.
And his withdrawal contributes to the dissatisfying sex life that
made you feel doubt in the first place.

Before you assume your husband wants to "play for the other
team," how about you pitch him some easier balls first and see
what happens? Consider other possibilities and ask him about
those. Come back to this option if other indicators point you here,
but not as a knee-jerk reaction to his lack of drive.

What If He Is Gay?

Ultimately, you need to cultivate the kind of safe atmosphere in
which your husband can confess whatever's holding him back.
That's great advice for all causes that could contribute to a man
having little to no sexual desire for his wife, but particularly important when the revelation is a game changer like this one.

Let's imagine you discover—through your own perceptiveness
or your husband's admission—that your husband isn't attracted
to women. What should you do?

I can't answer that question for you. Some couples part ways. Some couples remain married and focus on the friendship instead. Some couples work together to foster romantic or sexual interest in one another. What you choose to do depends on your life circumstances and religious ethics.

If you find yourself in this situation, I definitely recommend counseling to process what you've been through and what to do next. Choose a counselor who shares your values and can help you navigate the challenging journey ahead. May God give you wisdom.

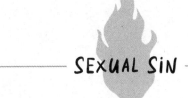

SEXUAL SIN

While sex was not a welcome topic in the church when I was growing up, sexual sin was. Yet even with periodic mentions of adultery, most of the *gasp*, "don't do that" content focused on making sure you didn't ruin it all by having sex before marriage. Which meant our Christian community wasn't wholly aligned with God's view of and commands about sex. And we failed to address issues that many Christians struggled with. Our silence about other sexual sin served to make people reluctant to get help, more likely to remain in their sin, and even leave the church altogether.

But I love how Christ Community Church of Denton explained one of their goals—that the church should be a safe place for sinners but a dangerous place for sin.

In this section, we'll address how sexual sin may have impacted your husband's sex drive and how we can make our marriage a safe place for sinners and a dangerous place for sin.

22. Extramarital Sex

When HDWs describe their husband's absence of sexual interest, others often respond with, "Maybe he's getting it somewhere else." Usually, that comment comes from someone who has only experienced a higher drive husband / lower drive wife scenario, and they can't imagine why a man wouldn't want more sex. Adultery is rarely the reason for a man having less sexual interest in his wife.

But now and then, it is.

Signs of an Affair

How can you know if he's cheating? Other than finding him in bed with another woman or encountering a text from him to another woman saying something like, "Thanks for the great sex last night," you can't know. Without direct evidence, you're picking up signals that make you think he's been busy elsewhere.

Experts identify several factors that could indicate an extramarital relationship, with *change* being the big factor:

- His personal routines change, from grooming to dieting to a shift in his schedule.
- His sex drive changes, taking a nosedive or becoming more insistent and even aggressive.

- His use of digital technology changes, with spending more time on social media or messaging, changing passwords to lock you out, or downloading apps.
- His spending habits change, with charges at places he didn't go before or shutting off your access to his accounts.
- His communication changes, from picking fights to stone-walling to making extra efforts to maintain peace.[1]

None of these alone screams, "I'm cheating!" But a few factors taken together could mean something's up and it's time to probe for answers.

Confronting Your Husband

If you think he's cheating, what can you do? Many wives confront their husband with their suspicion or evidence. Before you do that, check out wise resources that can advise you on how to proceed, such as Daring Ventures, Renewing Us Recovery, and Affair Recovery.

While I'm no expert in marital infidelity, I know quite a bit about HDWs and LDHs, so let me caution you not to accuse your husband of cheating based solely on his lack of sex drive. No woman should ignore her husband's infidelity, but she also shouldn't make false accusations simply because he isn't running to the bedroom with a huge grin and a "yeehaw!" every time she wants. Such erroneous finger wagging might make a husband shut down even more. Instead, examine the signs calmly, consider alternative explanations, seek the advice of a trusted resource, and proceed with clearheadedness.

If you then discover he is cheating, you're allowed to lose your cool. Who wouldn't?

But while you have every right to your anger, you should also proceed carefully. Feel the feels, but act with the good of your family in mind and with a clean conscience before God. Again, check out the ministries mentioned above for wise counsel.

Why Do Men Cheat?

For most men who engage in infidelity, the reasons are far more about their personal baggage and inattention to the marriage than about their wife. Feeling emotionally vulnerable in one way or another, and not feeling they can get their needs met through their marriage (whether or not that's true), such men become bull's-eye targets for Satan's temptation.

Every spouse should revisit Proverbs 5 from time to time to remind themselves of the wise father's warning against adultery, especially verses 15–21:

> Drink water from your own cistern,
>   running water from your own well.
> Should your springs overflow in the streets,
>   your streams of water in the public squares?
> Let them be yours alone,
>   never to be shared with strangers.
> May your fountain be blessed,
>   and may you rejoice in the wife of your youth.
> A loving doe, a graceful deer—
>   may her breasts satisfy you always,
>   may you ever be intoxicated with her love.
> Why, my son, be intoxicated with another man's wife?
>   Why embrace the bosom of a wayward woman?
> For your ways are in full view of the LORD,
>   and he examines all your paths.

This wisdom isn't convicting for everyone. Some cheaters are selfish liars and will cheat pretty much no matter what. These adulterers rarely show remorse for cheating; rather, they're upset about getting caught. Or they'll say, "Yes, I cheated," but then blame their spouse for their sin, as if their faithful mate drove them into the arms of their adulterer. If you're in this situation, I strongly suggest you meet with a licensed therapist and talk through how to handle a toxic person. Some toxic people change, but some won't.

However, if you have a husband who massively screwed up and knows it, you may be able to not only revive your marriage and sexual intimacy but rebuild an even better relationship. But that will take time, and you need to focus on first things first.

Begin by giving yourself space to feel your feelings, grieve this terrible loss, and cry out to God. He understands what it's like to love someone who is unfaithful (see Jer. 3:20; Hosea 1:2).

While still lamenting the emotional pain of your husband's betrayal, seek help to figure out what's next. You may want to seek out a marriage counselor for you both or start with a counselor for yourself. If you remain in the marriage, you'll need to set some boundaries and work toward rebuilding trust. All of this can happen better with the support of a counselor, coach, or ministry that understands your situation.

Many marriages have recovered from infidelity, but it is a long-term endeavor. Those who find safety and intimacy on the other side believe it's worth it, but make your own choices with the well-being of yourself and your family in mind, and in coordination with mentors who can help you navigate this struggle.

23. Pornography

A few years ago, Aria married a man who'd had a promiscuous past but (presumably) recommitted to God. However, porn had already altered his desires and expectations. "I kind of assumed that it had been a past thing just because of his lifestyle prior to meeting me, but I didn't know until a couple of years—probably at least three years into marriage—that he was still occasionally watching it, and now I don't even know . . . I don't know how often he watches it."

Aria suspects his sexual interest would be higher if she was willing to go along with his porn-inspired fantasies, such as threesomes. Wisely, she does not go along.

She aches for her husband to pursue true intimacy, rather than the counterfeit version promoted by pornography. If only he could open his mind and heart to what God wants this couple to have!

The Impact of Porn

Many wives relate to Aria's story. While porn has been with us from ancient times, only in recent years has it become so widely available that a simple click can drop titillating images onto your screen. And the sheer number of images makes variety and novelty not a perk but a given.

Some men react by becoming hypersexual. Their appetites become ravenous, and they hunger for more frequent sex with a real partner. Additionally, they may seek out a variety of experiences, pursuing the next adrenaline high like sex is an extreme sport.

Other men react by shutting down. They lose their appetite for sex with a real partner, preferring self-pleasure. Masturbation almost always accompanies pornography viewing, and since the feedback loop of pleasuring oneself is shorter than sex with a partner, it can become the preferred method for reaching climax. Also, sexual arousal may become connected to deviant activities seen in porn, and a husband doesn't want to act those out with the spouse he views with greater honor.

Neither reaction is healthy, for the person or the marriage. But if your lower desire husband is watching porn, he's in that second category: sexually avoidant. Let's look deeper into the problems with porn and what you can do if your husband's using it.

Has He Viewed Porn?

No matter who your husband is, it's 99% likely that he's seen pornography. While I grew up in a world where you had to seek out porn, these days you have to block out porn. Even a web search for something fairly innocent can bring up a slew of images you didn't bargain for.

We're exposed to all kinds of temptations in life, and being in the presence of sin doesn't make you a sinner. If your husband has seen porn, that makes him a normal person in a broken world. If your husband used porn in the past but walked away out of sexual integrity, then praise be to God! But if he got sucked into the vortex of vulgarity, he's not alone.

A 2014 survey commissioned by Proven Men Ministries and conducted by the Barna Group noted that over half (55%) of married men view pornography at least monthly, and 18% of all men surveyed thought they might be addicted to pornography or were unsure if they were addicted.[1] In a separate 2017 report, Barna noted, "Most pastors (57%) and youth pastors (64%) admit they have struggled with porn, either currently or in the past."[2]

While every man does not get swept away by the temptation of pornography or lust, too many do. Is your husband one of them?

Maybe you know your husband views porn or suspect he does. Maybe you have no idea whether he's engaged with porn. Sometimes the only sign that he's viewing it is his lack of interest in sex with you. Since low sex drive can be caused by many things, pornography isn't necessarily the reason.

But sometimes it is.

Porn Can Deflate His Desire, Literally

Several years back, doctors and researchers began noticing that young men lacked the sexual interest previous generations had, and high exposure to porn seemed to account not only for that disinterest but also for some men's inability to achieve erections with real-world partners. Experts named this phenomenon porn-induced erectile dysfunction, or PIED.

Since then, some studies have shown a correlation of high porn use and erectile dysfunction, while others have indicated a correlation only when the user feels bad about viewing porn. Indeed, several secular experts go to great lengths to suggest that the problem people should be concerned about isn't porn use, which some sex therapists even recommend to clients, but rather societal strictures that make a porn user feel shame.

Being a Christian, I believe one *should* feel guilty about sinning—enough to repent and seek forgiveness. Porn use does not honor God's design for sexuality, marriage, or people. And even many who don't agree with me on that have noted the link between using porn and difficulty with arousal in a relationship.

In an online article, Dr. Robert Weiss, who runs treatment centers for male sexual addicts and their families, identifies typical signs of porn-conditioned male sexual dysfunction as follows:

- A man is able to get hard and have orgasms with porn, but he struggles with real world partners.
- A man is able to have sex with real world partners, but orgasm takes a long time.
- A man's real world partners complain that he seems disengaged during lovemaking (typically because he's replaying clips of porn in his mind as a way to stay hard and reach orgasm).
- A man says he prefers porn sex to real world sex, finding online imagery more arousing and intense than an in-the-flesh partner.[3]

Do any of those descriptions sound familiar?

Porn may or may not be involved in the disparity between your sex drive and your husband's, but as you consider that possibility, it's worth recognizing that ongoing porn use can make it more difficult for many men to perform physically. But an uncooperative penis is just one negative result of porn use.

Porn Warps Our View of Sexuality

If you're looking for a Bible verse that says, "Don't look at naked people for your own sexual pleasure," you won't find it. But we don't need specific verses against this practice. Rather, "the whole counsel of God" (Acts 20:27 ESV)—that is, the Word of God studied in full—screams against the use of porn.

Genesis 2:24 proclaims, "That is why a man leaves his father and mother and is united to his wife, and they become one flesh." The first time sexual intercourse is recorded, the Bible says, "Adam *knew* Eve his wife" (Gen. 4:1 ESV, emphasis added). Many translations now use "had relations" or "made love," but the original Hebrew word is *yada*, which connotes really knowing someone. Terms like "one flesh" and "knew" give us a foundational understanding of God's design for sex as an intimate act in the context of marriage.

Now go look at all the passages about sexual sin. I'll wait.

Never mind, that could take weeks! How about I summarize? The long and short of it is that whenever someone exploits another for their sexual pleasure, it's condemned. You won't find any positive coverage of people who lusted, coveted, or sexually used others. God's image bearers are not sex toys.

Yet pornography treats them that way. In porn, "actors" pose, parade, and perform for money or power, and sexual acts are a product intended to arouse and satisfy the consumer. Meanwhile, the consumer doesn't have to put forth any response to the person turning him (or her) on. He or she can arrive in any state and still receive the same product. Moreover, it's not one product but many the consumer can choose from—many people, many contexts, many acts, many taboo desires, and more. Sex becomes all about the consumer and his or her choices, devaluing the other participant and reducing the experience to an impersonal transaction.

Intimate sex with a loving spouse is so much better. But it's also a more difficult journey. If porn is a shortcut, mutually satisfying sex with a real person is a hike through the mountains—gorgeous scenery but challenging trails. Men regularly engaging with pornography—and the masturbation that almost always accompanies it—may expend their sexual energy outside the marriage bed, leaving little to nothing to offer their wife.

But that's not the only problem. These men also adopt a wholly unrealistic view of sexuality. It may be disheartening for a man primed by porn to discover that a woman requires longer to become aroused, doesn't want to engage in certain sexual acts, and longs for greater romance and connection. Logically, he might see the benefit of all that, but porn has worn grooves of erroneous expectations into his brain, and he can't seem to move beyond them.

Kristen's husband came into marriage with a porn addiction. While he's worked on overcoming it, she noted, "He's admitted to me before, 'sex is just not as exciting as I thought it was going to be.'"

Porn creates perverse notions about what good sex is and requires.

But I'm Here!

In far too many Christian circles, men who look at porn blame their wives, claiming they turned to this vice when they were sexually shut off by their spouse. That argument is bunk, no matter what.

And that's not your story. You may have read that accusation and thought, *But I'm here! Ready and willing!* Why on earth would a husband choose porn over a willing wife?

First, porn use nearly always predates the marriage, often by a long time. Bonny Burns is my cohost on our podcast, *Sex Chat for Christian Wives*, and an APSATS-certified coach who works with sexually betrayed wives. She shared, "In every one of my cases, childhood is where porn use started."[4] Statistics back this up, with a Common Sense Media survey of over a thousand teens, ages 13–17, reporting the average age for first viewing pornography was 12 years, and 15% first saw online pornography at age 10 or younger.[5] How many 10- to 12-year-olds can be expected to handle such exposure well?

If they don't see it by 12 years old, it's coming. In their 2016 study, Barna reported, "Nearly three-quarters of young adults (71%) and half of teens (50%) come across what they consider to be porn at least once a month, whether they are seeking it or not."[6]

While some young people stop after that first view, many others fall into a rabbit hole and find themselves drawn into a world they didn't quite understand when they began viewing porn. Some are simply curious, but for those with an emotional wound—"a negative experience, or series of experiences, that causes pain on a deep psychological level"[7]—the effect can be devastating. They begin to lean on pornography as a self-soothing coping mechanism, and by the time they enter adulthood, breaking free can feel like trying to step out of a spinning hurricane.

As part of her work with sexually betrayed wives, Bonny Burns has often been present when a husband confesses his ongoing porn use to a wife, including how his sexual past influenced his current problem. Bonny has this message to wives whose husbands are steeped in porn:

> It's not about you. In disclosure after disclosure after disclosure that I've been in, the reason we asked the guys to start their sexual history from the first time they remember anything sexual is so that she will see this has nothing to do with you. He brings it in with him.[8]

A man's childhood wound likely has more to do with persistent porn use than anything a wife has done or could do. While you have every reason to be angry if he's been diverting sexual energy away from you to porn, you might discover some compassion alongside that anger if you can imagine the young boy your husband once was, wounded by life, exposed to pornography, and pulled into this odious world of sin and shame.

Speaking of which, a second point: while feelings of guilt or shame should motivate us to seek help and pursue healthier sexuality, many Christian men go the opposite way—hiding in the shadows and praying that others, especially their wife, don't find out. The paradox is that such a burden weighs him down further, pushing him into the very conditions that make him reach for his (awful) coping mechanism.

A lower desire husband who comes up with every excuse in the book could be concealing a porn habit or addiction. He may brush off your questions, avoid eye contact when talking about sex, or complain about you pushing the issue without you being pushy in the least. All to keep the secret he's scared to share.

A third reason your husband might avoid sexual intimacy is that, as I pointed out before, porn is easier. Sex with a real partner requires more from a man than an image or video. After discussing the selfish nature of porn, I suggested to Bonny that men might pursue porn out of sexual laziness. She had a different take:

> I think it's more fear. . . . Even if he's got a higher drive wife, [he may be thinking,] what if I am rejected? And it's just those childhood scripts that he hasn't navigated. . . . Scripts are what we tell ourselves to try to explain what's happening in our world, and in childhood, they often carry self-blame or shame as well as survival techniques that serve us well in the moment but set us up for problems in future relationships. For instance, if a man had a mother who mocked him when he expressed emotion, he may enter marriage believing that he can't be emotionally vulnerable or he'll get hurt. Given that experience, his attachment style—the type of bond one has with their primary caregiver that's usually taken into future relationships—may be anxious or avoidant. Both of which come from not feeling secure.[9]

Your husband's avoidance might strike you as foolish, given how much you've indicated your desire, willingness to engage, and satisfaction with sexual activity in marriage. But again, it's not about you. He's hung up on bad scripts in his mind, and giving up the crutch—even for a far better experience—feels too risky or even impossible.

Fourth, porn feeds the cycle again and again and again. Our brains reward us for feel-good activities with dopamine hits, and porn hijacks that system to provide pleasure pings that keep viewers coming back. Meanwhile, the content of porn makes many men feel inadequate, from well-endowed actors to actresses who dramatically overreact to whatever the actor does on-screen. Since a husband can't match that experience in real life, why even try? And racked with guilt or shame, he turns back to the one avenue for his sexuality that feeds his distorted need for affirmation—pornography. It's a loop of lies too many husbands can't seem to leave.

Porn Isn't Just a Man's Game

Men aren't the only ones using porn. Some higher desire wives have turned to pornography as a place to sate their desire, while others discovered a high or higher drive after fueling their libido with pornographic content—whether strictly XXX or highly erotic imagery and prose.

Years ago, one wife wrote me to explain that her higher drive had kicked in after she'd read *Fifty Shades of Grey*. Having become aroused by fictional scenes of BDSM, she wanted her husband to play those out in their bedroom. Despite my efforts to encourage her otherwise, she continued to insist that erotica had been good for her sexuality. Within a short time, she dropped off commenting on my and colleagues' blogs, and I've often wondered if she's still married. She wasn't treating her husband as an intimate partner but rather as a tool for her sexual pleasure.

If you're using pornography, please recognize the damage you're doing to your marriage and your soul. God loves you and wants you to break free, but you likely need help. Reach out to get the support you need. Two well-established ministries that help women involved in pornography are SheRecovery and Beggar's Daughter.

What If Your Husband Is into Porn?

If you're not sure, don't go spying on him. Even as I type that, I feel like I'd have a terrible time not spying on my husband if I thought he was choosing porn over me. Not only am I a perpetually curious person, I was raised on Nancy Drew, *Columbo*, and

Charlie's Angels. I'm a huuuuge *Veronica Mars* fan. If I thought my husband was engaging with porn, I would want to know.

But I refer and defer to those who know, and I'll cite sexual betrayal coach Bonny Burns again:

> It's a violation, and you're acting outside of your own values. That's where it lands. You've got to know what your values are and continue to act in them, even if you're triggered, the best you can.[10]

Bonny identifies several red flags that may indicate your husband is hiding porn use:

- a hard resistance to turn on location sharing, such as the Google Maps tracker or Life360
- pushback about using filtering software for the whole family, including him
- an unwillingness to share passwords or phone history

She encourages wives to engage in calm conversations and prayer, especially focused on Luke 8:17: "For there is nothing hidden that will not be disclosed, and nothing concealed that will not be known or brought out into the open." If you believe your husband is using porn, pray and pursue the truth while acknowledging that revelation won't lead to change unless and until he's ready.

A recovering husband explained it to me this way: "I quit nineteen times because I was caught, and once for me."

That's discouraging, right? Yeah, I know.

The number one question I get is "How can I make my spouse _____?" Whatever you put in that blank, the answer is the same: you can't. You can't *make* your spouse do anything. But you do have a lot of influence.

In their book *Boundaries,* Christian psychologists Henry Cloud and John Townsend show how we can set calm, firm boundaries about what we will and won't do in our relationships, both to protect ourselves and to encourage change in others. Jesus Christ himself set boundaries by welcoming people at some times but stepping away at others, knowing he needed to maintain his emotional health and spiritual focus.

To say yes to the sexual intimacy God designed, we must say no to the counterfeits. If your husband has denied your marriage the physical intimacy it deserves due to porn use, what boundaries will you set? Once again, the book *Boundaries* can guide you.

Is There Hope?

I'm not the most optimistic person. I'm a skeptic at best, a pessimist more often. My mind automatically goes to what could go wrong and mucks around in that sludge for a while before remembering that Christ already won the victory. So when I say this next thing, don't imagine some smiling motivational speaker trying to get you to believe the impossible.

Things can get better. If I shared the stories of all the couples who came through a pornography habit, compulsion, or addiction and now have a genuinely intimate marriage with mutually fulfilling sex, this book would rival the length of a George R. R. Martin novel. (He's the guy who wrote *A Game of Thrones*, and his books are notoriously long.)

Also, there are many resources now devoted to helping couples navigate this tricky situation. From my friend Bonny Burns coaching wives who've been sexually betrayed, to sites like Proven Men, Covenant Eyes, and Fight the New Drug, to online ministries like Samson Society, Be Broken, and Pure Desire Ministries, to local ministries like Bethesda Workshops, you can find help and hope.

Many marriages thrive after the discovery of persistent porn use and subsequent healing. If you think this is an issue in your marriage, speak calmly with your husband and learn more about unwanted sexual behavior. Above all, pray that all will be revealed and your husband will be convicted to come clean and find healing.

24. Sexual Acting Out

This chapter builds on the last one, since most of the time, those who act out sexual fantasies started with pornography. Aroused by sexual imagery, some shift from passive viewer to active participant—like going to strip clubs and getting lap dances, visiting "massage parlors" that do far more than therapeutic massage, sex chatting with women online or by phone, or hiring a prostitute.

Once again, two options arise from such sexual acting out:

- a husband becomes even more sexually intense with his wife, his appetite roused but never satisfied
- a husband becomes less engaged with his wife, his appetite gone after getting fed elsewhere or shut down by shame

Since you're reading this book, I suspect you're not experiencing the former but rather a husband who's less engaged. Could it be due to sexual acting out? Let's talk more about what sexual acting out involves.

What's Going On?

In 2009, professional golfer Tiger Woods was exposed as a serial cheater whose escapades involved mistresses, porn stars, strippers, and escorts. I recall the news coverage, specifically how his wife chased him out of the house with a golf club, and frankly, I thought that was fair. Soon after, Woods checked into a sexual addiction clinic, and media outlets turned toward the issue of sexual addiction—what is it, how does it manifest, is it even real?

There's an ongoing debate about whether sexual acting out (and persistent porn use) qualifies as a habit, an addiction, or a compulsion. On one hand, persistent porn use and more extreme behaviors mirror substance addiction in important ways:

- A person tries it out of curiosity or intrigue.
- Their body delivers a natural chemical reward.
- They seek out stronger forms of the substance to receive the same or a more intense effect.
- They experience a mix of good feelings and bad consequences.
- If they try to quit, they may experience resistance or a sense of loss.[1]

However, sexual acting out doesn't have the same effect on the body as substance addiction. With a smoking addiction, for instance, nicotine stimulates acetylcholine and causes the release of glutamate—both neurochemicals that provide extra-good feelings.[2] When your brain doesn't get the chemicals it has become used to having, you can experience physiological withdrawal. With sexual acting out, the main brain chemical implicated is dopamine, often known as the feel-good hormone, which releases whenever something good happens, including sex with your spouse. So our brains don't activate quite the same way with sexual acting out and substance addiction.

Many suggest that sexual acting out is more like a compulsion. A compulsion is a behavior engaged in repeatedly to reduce anxiety or distress, often one that's troubling or interferes with normal functioning. Yes, it could be washing your hands over and over, but it could also be excessive gambling or sexual acting out. The World Health Organization characterized sexual acting out in their most recent International Classification of Diseases (ICD-11) as Compulsive Sexual Behavior Disorder, or CSBD.[3]

Some prefer instead to call it a bad habit. It could be that as well. Consider this description of how we develop habits:

- A person forms a habit through a system of cue/trigger, routine, and reward. For instance, the smell of coffee (cue) leads them to drink coffee (routine) and feel a reward (yum and more energy).
- They reinforce the behavior through repetition.
- Anticipating the reward, they feel a craving for the routine.
- They subconsciously link the habit to other environmental triggers (for example, a certain room or time of day).
- Even when the habit is hurting them (or people they love), they fall back on the entrenched routine.[4]

That's a quick overview of how addictions, habits, and compulsions form, and you may lean toward one particular label. But in the end, does it matter what it's called? No. Sexual acting out is destructive to the person engaging in it and those he loves.

Delving Deeper

Whether it's an addiction, compulsion, or habit, someone engaging in this unwanted sexual behavior feels trapped. They're participating in these actions willfully but without a full sense of control. Making the right choice involves fighting back against a whole system of trigger-routine-reward that screams at them to continue.

For some, labeling it an addiction or compulsion encourages them to seek the outside help they need. They no longer feel they must white-knuckle their way to the other side but recognize this problem is bigger than they thought and they need reinforcements to fight their way out.

For others, the addiction or compulsion label makes them feel let off the hook for their choices and perhaps even for changing their behaviors. "I can't help it, it's an addiction" is not what any rejected wife wants to hear. Yes, your husband may need and benefit from the support of others, but he can't blame a label for his misdeeds. If the word "addiction" or "compulsion" keeps him from doing what he should to stop acting out sexually, then talking about habits and behaviors could prove more productive.

If you think your husband is engaged in sexual acting out, remember that his behavior is not about you. Of course, it feels like it's about you. After all, you've been there, willing to have sex, wanting to be physically connected, and yet he's going off and engaging in sexual stuff with others but not you. How can that not feel personal?

But these problems likely predated you. Christian therapist Jay Stringer has engaged in therapy with many men and women involved in unwanted sexual behavior and has seen vast evidence that "the formative experiences of our childhood (loneliness, pain, sexual arousal, secrecy, and relational ambivalence) are all being repeated in our unwanted sexual behavior as adults."[5] Even if your husband started acting out only after marriage, he came into the marriage with all the deep-seated issues that made him turn to these behaviors as coping mechanisms, ways to reduce anxiety and distress.

These attempts to self-soothe don't last. They lead to feeling even more hollow and needy than before and, soon enough, a longing for the next "hit."

What Can You Do?

As tempting as it is to chase him out of the house with a golf club—oh so tempting—I encourage you to get help yourself to figure out how the unwanted sexual behavior came about, what it's done to your husband's mind and his sexuality, and the best way to navigate this situation with your husband. Jay Stringer's book *Unwanted* or Eddie Capparucci's book *Going Deeper* could clarify what brought your husband to this point.

Of course, you should ask him to stop these vile, destructive behaviors. But knowing that sheer will likely won't be enough, you can explain why he needs to seek help through a licensed counselor or support group. If he's not eager for that (yet), you could suggest reading one of the books mentioned above together or simply watching a video from Jay Stringer on YouTube on the topic. Asking for action on his part may need to be followed up with a boundary of what you will do to maintain your emotional safety if he doesn't take appropriate action.

What boundaries are right for you in your marriage? Well, this is not a journey you should white-knuckle your way through either. Find someone who works with sexually betrayed partners, such as an APSATS-trained counselor or coach or a Christian support group for wives who've experienced betrayal trauma. They can help you determine how to proceed in a way that protects you, promotes healing for your husband, and—hopefully—produces a stronger marriage.

What if your husband is unrepentant? I'm not talking about the husband who seeks help, makes progress, then messes up again and feels remorse for his actions. Someone can stumble but still be on the right path. Rather, what about the husband who doesn't want to address his sexual acting out? I cannot decide that for you. But what I can say once again is that you need someone helping you walk through this valley of anguish. There's a reason it's called sexual betrayal, or simply infidelity. Find a pastor, mentor, or counselor who can help you be clear-eyed about your decision.

But if your husband is repentant and willing to seek help, you can get through this. It won't be easy, but many couples have come through it, established healthy boundaries, and discovered loving, respectful sexual intimacy as God intended.

Your Relationship

Almost every Christian marriage resource speaks as if marriage is made up of a higher desire husband and a lower desire wife and encourages men to attend more to the relationship. The advice goes something like this: *Romance and cherish her, partner with her on household management and parenting, show affection even when you're initiating sex, and love her for who she is, not just what she offers in the bedroom.*

These resources rightly address that many women lose sexual interest when their marriage isn't healthy. And yet, little attention is paid to the fact that many husbands also shut down sexually when the relationship isn't going well. Your husband may be one of them. If things aren't positive in your marriage, he may feel negative about having sex.

As we've discussed, truly intimate sex requires trusting your partner with your body and your heart in this vulnerable experience. So of course the relationship matters! Let's talk about a few aspects of it.

25. Lack of Attraction

When a husband isn't interested in sex, his wife can quickly leap to the conclusion that she's unappealing to him. Why would he avoid getting turned on *with* her unless he was turned off *by* her?

HDWs often take stock of their appearance, look for flaws, and conclude that maybe it's their weight or their breast size or their height or their butt or their [name a physical trait] that poses the problem. If only she looked like that actress he likes or that magazine model he caught a glimpse of, then maybe he'd be raring to go.

Only rarely is that what's happening. And even when appearance is part of the equation, it's typically not her appearance itself but other factors at play.

Am I Pretty?

In Song of Songs, the husband declares to his wife, "You are altogether beautiful, my darling; there is no flaw in you" (4:7). His compliment is even more significant when you consider that she previously pointed out a flaw she saw in herself: "Do not stare at me because I am dark, because I am darkened by the sun. My mother's sons were angry with me and made me take care of the vineyards; my own vineyard I had to neglect" (1:6). For the rest of the book, she never again downplays her appearance.

His reassurance that she's perfect to him and for him settled her heart so that she could be vulnerable and intimate with her beloved.

Just reading that, you probably had a lot of thoughts. Maybe about how you wish that was your husband's attitude. Maybe about how you were misled to believe that your husband would feel that way. Maybe about grabbing a pint of Häagen-Dazs ice cream and ignoring the "serves 4" label on the package—after all, if he doesn't think you're pretty enough, what's the point?

Over and over I hear from HDWs that their husband's lack of interest results in them not feeling desired or desirable. But is that what a husband's lower sex drive means?

What Turns Him Off?

A husband wrote me about his three years with an unconsummated marriage. Among several issues he named, he shared this about his wife:

> I'm not attracted to her at all. I never have been. . . . Basically everyone I knew and respected pushed for us to date because we were similar in many ways and had similar interests. Over time I started to think maybe I was being selfish or vain for wanting to date someone I was attracted to and conceded to date. I knew the attraction piece was totally missing, but friends and family pushed so hard that I doubted myself and we got engaged.

He named physical attributes that were unappealing to him, but they centered less on her appearance than her approach. It wasn't that she was obese, but she didn't want to get healthy. It wasn't that she didn't wear makeup, but she wouldn't use anything that might emphasize her best features. It wasn't that she didn't wear what he would have liked, but she didn't bother to dress well at all. Putting it all together, it seemed that he was supposed to be attracted to the appearance of someone who cared little to nothing about her appearance.

Of course, a husband can influence how a wife feels about herself. If he treats her as someone with beauty and value, she may believe it more herself and make greater efforts to put her best foot, or face, forward. Moreover, no wife should feel that she must be "on" at all times. She should be appreciated when she looks ready to walk the Oscars red carpet and when she's wearing sweats, gardening gloves, and half the dirt from their flower beds.

But as I communicated with this husband, it reminded me that how appealing you find your spouse often has less to do with objective physical features and more with how they present themselves. Do they attend to basic grooming? Do they pursue good health? Do they show off their good traits by how they dress, style their hair, or even sit in a chair? (Posture matters, y'all. It really does.)

After I sent him suggestions on helping his wife feel her value, he wrote me another email in which he acknowledged he was put off by her view of herself more than her appearance. He longed for his wife to feel confident about her beauty and to act accordingly. We'll talk about that confidence in a bit, but first, this question: what features do men find attractive?

What Makes a Woman Appealing?

As part of the extensive research done for this book, I asked my husband, "What makes a woman sexy?" Though he's a man of few words, his answer tracked with what I've heard from many men over the course of my ministry: "Curves, being clean, a smile, kind words."

Sure, the airbrushed model in the Victoria's Secret window looks good, but that's not what a good husband typically wants for his wife. He's taken by her curves, her personality, her love for him. He wants her to care for herself, feel confident, and have good character. As the apostle Peter instructed wives,

Your adornment must not be merely the external—braiding the
hair, wearing gold jewelry, or putting on apparel; but it should be
the hidden person of the heart, with the imperishable quality of
a gentle and quiet spirit, which is precious in the sight of God.
(1 Peter 3:3–4 NASB)

By the way, I used to think "gentle and quiet spirit" meant that
women who spoke boldly, laughed loudly, or otherwise didn't
comport with the idea of a soft-spoken, polite lady didn't meet
biblical beauty requirements. But that's not what the phrase
means. The New Testament Greek adjective for "gentle" is
praus, and the noun form is *prautes*. The noun form shows
that a gentle spirit is about kindness rather than harshness. For
example:

What do you prefer? Shall I come to you with a rod of discipline,
or shall I come in love and with a *gentle* spirit? (1 Cor. 4:21, emphasis added)

Brothers and sisters, if someone is caught in a sin, you who live by
the Spirit should restore that person *gently*. But watch yourselves,
or you also may be tempted. (Gal. 6:1, emphasis added)

Let your *gentleness* be evident to all. The Lord is near. (Phil. 4:5,
emphasis added)

While caring for our appearance matters, kindness and goodness can make or break how we appear to others. Including our
husband.

An Attractive Package

Among other challenges they faced, Naomi noted that her words
often came across to her husband as criticism. He even recounted
to her a conversation he once had with a friend: "I told him I don't

want sex when I don't feel loved by my wife." Naomi wisely noted, "I really don't think it's like, oh, men want sex to feel loved"—a common statement in many Christian circles. "I think men want to feel loved."

Our positive traits combined with our feminine forms make for an attractive package. But true beauty is about who we are, not just what we present.

Could there be something about your inner character, your care for yourself, or your harshness with your husband that, unwittingly, turns him off?

Again, you don't need to be a perfect specimen of womanhood. Indeed, feeling good about yourself is an attractive quality. But even if it weren't, it's good for your soul to embrace how God created you, your body as it exists today, and the beauty you embody just by being *you*. Regardless of whether your husband appreciates your efforts, you should care for yourself, understand your worth as God's artwork, and be confident about all the positive qualities you bring to your marriage . . . and hey, the world!

Feeling Good About Your Appearance

I have a whole blog series on my website dedicated to helping women feel beautiful. I wrote some of the posts, but guest writers also came on and shared their tips. Much of what we wrote about came down to a few key issues.

First, remind yourself that the images that set beauty standards are fake. The models on magazines are made up, dressed up, and airbrushed. The actresses on the red carpet have shapewear underneath their dresses, went through plastic surgery, and/or can afford a personal chef and fitness trainer. Social media influencers use specific lighting, certain angles, or a camera filter to look better. Media encourages us to set unrealistic expectations of ourselves, and we should resist. Supermodel Cindy Crawford famously noted that her own images didn't represent reality: "I think women see me on the cover of magazines and think I never have a pimple or bags under my eyes. You have to realize that's after two hours of hair and makeup, plus retouching. Even I don't wake up looking like Cindy Crawford."[1]

Second, appreciate your body for what it can do. Our bodies don't exist to be looked at but to be utilized. Tap into gratitude for how God enables your body to do everything from walking with those great legs of yours to smiling with that lovely mouth to holding your children or husband with your soft arms. Move your body more to feel its efficacy. Pay attention to your five senses and how they serve you not only to get things done but to appreciate the world around you, like the scent of a flower, the taste of dessert, and the feel of your husband's hand. Lean into recognizing that you are "awesomely and wonderfully made" (Ps. 139:14 NASB).

Third, identify which of your physical features you believe are attractive. Too many women, when asked what they like about their appearance, can't come up with more than one or two items. But each woman possesses beauty, and noting what's beautiful about ourselves can help us feel more confident. For instance, I like my legs, my dimples, and the color of my eyes. Once I identified these as positive features, I paid more attention to them when looking in the mirror, I looked for ways to show them off, and I was motivated to identify more good parts of myself. Challenge yourself to come up with only three items, as I first did, but then increase that over time so that you end up with lots about yourself to like.

Fourth, practice self-care. It's easy to put yourself last when your workplace, your family, your household, and your friends all need something from you. But you're likely to be far more effective and confident in life if you take some time for yourself. Care for your body and your appearance as best you can in the season you're in. You may not have time for the full spa day you'd love, but you can probably grab a few minutes for a bubble bath, a half hour for the haircut you've been putting off, or an hour for the fitness class you've wanted to attend. Reasonable self-care isn't selfishness but good stewardship of the body God gave you.

Finally, just tell yourself you're pretty. That seems simplistic, but positive self-talk works. You can memorize verses to recite when not feeling great about yourself, such as Psalm 139:13–14:

> For you created my inmost being;
> > you knit me together in my mother's womb.
> I praise you because I am fearfully and wonderfully made;
> > your works are wonderful,
> I know that full well.

Or perhaps Proverbs 31:25: "She is clothed with strength and dignity; she can laugh at the days to come."

Go through that list of features you like that we talked about above. Ask what you would tell a friend who isn't feeling attractive, and then be a friend to yourself and provide that encouragement. We tend to believe what we tell ourselves over and over, so why not tell yourself the truth? You are a beautiful woman made in the image of God.

But What If . . . ?

What if, despite your inherent beauty and care for yourself, your husband really isn't attracted to you? I hate to say it, but yeah, some guys don't have sex with their wives because they don't like how she looks. Even though she looks absolutely fine.

If that's your situation, then know it's not about you. It's about his unrealistic expectations, his shallow perception of beauty, his selfish desires, and his perspective of women as eye candy. Where that viewpoint came from, I can't say. Perhaps it's from his own sexual brokenness—it often is—but whatever the source, that perspective objectifies women in terms of what they do for *him* rather than viewing a woman on her own terms.

Now, it may seem like I just described such men without using a "gentle and quiet spirit," but read what Peter said to husbands: "Husbands, in the same way be considerate as you live with your wives, and treat them with respect as the weaker partner and as heirs with you of the gracious gift of life, so that nothing will hinder your prayers" (1 Pet. 3:7).

So a lack of consideration and respect for one's wife can put a barrier between a husband and God? Apparently. And sharing that isn't harsh but rather a wake-up call.

Having that conversation with your husband may be worthwhile—explaining how his viewpoint makes you feel and how it's causing a wedge in your relationship as well. Pray for him to see things as God sees them. And take care of yourself—physically, emotionally, and spiritually—so that you will become comfortable in and confident of your sex appeal, whether or not your husband can see it yet.

26. Relational Tension

"It's not you, it's him." That's the premise of this section about what might be going on with your husband. But what if it's not him? What if it is you? At least partly.

Before you get defensive, let me share a personal story.

About ten years into my marriage, I genuinely thought we weren't going to make it. Things were terrible between my husband and me, and I didn't see how they could improve. I felt my husband wasn't listening to me, honoring my needs and desires, or partnering with me to make our marriage better. Why didn't he care as much as I did? Why did he shut down whenever I tried to work on our relationship?

Looking back, I can see that the way I expressed those feelings—with disrespect, harshness, and self-righteousness—made everything worse. Whether my complaints were legitimate or not, the criticism and contempt that seeped through my words and actions made my husband less willing to be with me and work with me.

My body could have been supermodel sexy—it wasn't, but let's pretend it was—but my behavior made me unattractive. I wouldn't have wanted to be married to me.

Sleeping with the Enemy

You may believe that more or better sex would draw you closer together and relieve the tension between you, but that might not work for your husband. When you're in relational conflict, distanced from one another, or highly critical, your husband may not see someone he's eager to sleep with. He may feel attacked or abandoned, and his heart screams to protect itself against this enemy.

Some men need to feel emotionally safe, respected, and desired to engage in the bedroom. Without those feelings, it may be difficult for your husband to want to even go there.

Tearing Down the House

Proverbs 14:1 warns, "The wise woman builds her house, but with her own hands the foolish one tears hers down."

Wait! you say. *I'm the one trying to build our house!*

Here's the thing: the foolish don't know they're being foolish. I didn't know. I thought I was right, and if only I could get my husband to see it—whatever that took—things would get good again. All the while, I was taking down brick after brick of our relationship.

I'm not saying he didn't have his own responsibility. If anything, husbands are called to greater responsibility, such as the command to "love your wives, just as Christ loved the church and gave himself up for her" (Eph. 5:25). But that doesn't absolve the wife for her part in adding to relational tension and conflict.

So, with a deep breath and deep humility, ask yourself how you've been tearing down your house. What if your husband spoke to you the way you speak to him? Or made the contemptuous facial expressions you've made? How about the actions or inactions you've engaged in that make your husband feel less valued?

Here's a reminder of who we should be in relation to others, including our husband:

The fruit of the Spirit is love, joy, peace, forbearance, kindness, goodness, faithfulness, gentleness and self-control. Against such things there is no law. (Gal. 5:22–23)

Love is patient, love is kind. It does not envy, it does not boast, it is not proud. It does not dishonor others, it is not self-seeking, it is not easily angered, it keeps no record of wrongs. Love does not delight in evil but rejoices with the truth. It always protects, always trusts, always hopes, always perseveres. (1 Cor. 13:4–7)

Does your treatment of your husband live up to the fruit of the Spirit or 1 Corinthians 13 love? Of course not. Nor does your husband's treatment of you. None of us lives up to that all the time. Thus the need for a Savior! But does your husband feel loved?

Owning Our Part

As previously mentioned, the most common question I receive is, "How can I make my spouse _____?" What's in that blank differs, but it's the same basic question with the same basic answer: you can't.

We have this thing called free will, gifted to us by God. So unless you're planning to hold your husband hostage and force him to comply on threat of violence or deprivation—surely not!—then all you've got is influence. You can't control him, and if you could, you'd lose respect for and interest in your now-puppet husband.

How, then, can you make things better? You work on yourself. You own your part of the problem, take your bad habits and sins to the Lord and ask for his transforming power, then little by little make healthy changes on yourself.

That's how my own marriage got vastly better. My husband certainly altered some of his attitudes and behaviors, but positive change began with me memorizing Galatians 5:22–23 and 1 Corinthians 13:4–7. Whenever I felt irritated or longed to lash out, I'd cite those verses in my head, reminding myself what characteristics I wanted to exhibit instead. Sometimes I didn't even get past "love is patient, love is kind" before realizing how I needed to alter my approach.

Even if your husband is 90% of the issue, your 10% can change the dynamic of your marriage. If you don't cooperate with bad-relationship behavior, then his game gets thrown off and he has to try something else. After a while, he may try those godly characteristics himself, especially as you are becoming healthier, holier, and happier—a magnetic combination.

Asking for Help

Many troubled relationships require or could benefit from outside support. If your struggles include any of the three A's—abuse, addiction, adultery—then you should seek professional help. But even with lesser difficulties, like different communication styles or marital expectations, a quality Christian counselor can help you reveal what's happening and learn how to address it.

Other options include mentors, support groups, marriage intensives, conferences or retreats, books, and classes. Don't expect a silver bullet. A single marriage weekend, reading a book or two, or a couple of visits with a therapist isn't going to fix everything. Healing is a process that takes work. But there's a lot of good information available that can help you and your husband get on the right track.

Once on that track, the two of you can ride it into a better relationship and more sparks between you.

27. And Baby Makes Three

Consider this tale: Once upon a time, he loved to look at you, to flirt with you, to initiate lovemaking with you, and to have sex with you. Then you got pregnant. Or maybe it was after the baby came. Perhaps it was while you nursed. Regardless, something shifted, and he no longer seemed nearly as interested.

If this is your story, you probably wondered whether your somewhat altered body made you unattractive to your husband. If so, would he ever want you again? And what did it convey about how much he really loved you if a big tummy, some stretch marks, or a couple of leaky breasts were deal-breakers?

It's perfectly reasonable to ask these kinds of questions if a shift in your husband's desire occurs after a baby enters the picture. But the situation is likely more complex.

Lover or Mother?

Many moms struggle to see themselves as a sexy lover. It happens for some while pregnant, as their body's shape and functions are taken over by a growing life inside, and they lose the figure they knew and shared with their husband. For others, it's after the child comes. They reach the end of the day exhausted and with spit-up or other signs of motherhood on their body, keep one eye and one ear open for the baby's cries, and feel overloaded from being touched all day long and thus are not eager for affection from their husband. Perhaps they even struggle with the idea of a mother doing the things involved in sex that they used to do. Are mamas allowed to be sexy?

Some husbands wonder that too. Their wife turning into a mother throws off their sexual compass. They find it hard to hold in their heads and hearts the two roles of lover and mother. They haven't lost their attraction to their wife. Indeed, it may be greater! But it's taken a different form—wonder for this life-sustaining woman that feels out of sync with their previous wonder of her super-sexy bod.

Husbands can also be overly sensitive in not wanting to do anything that could harm their wife or child. For instance, some men find it hard to have sex with their pregnant wife for fear of hurting the infant inside. Even if there's no cause for concern, they can't quite convince their muscles and nerves to relax and enjoy.

A husband may feel his role is to let the child have his wife's full attention, so his sexual desires should be back-burnered. Or he worries that sex too soon will hurt his wife's body, particularly because it's a different body from before that he's not quite used to. Again, this isn't a lack of attraction. He may think you're as hot as ever, but anxiety is calling the shots.

"But I'm a Dad"

Then there's the husband who feels the weight of fatherhood so intensely, he devotes far more time and attention to being a dad than a husband. This development is more likely after the infant years, when a child becomes more active and a father discovers the demands and joys of teaching life skills, coaching a team or leading a scout troop, or just engaging in play with and the care of a beloved child.

For some men, the father-child relationship is easier to navigate than the husband-wife relationship, so they lean into the former and neglect the latter. After all, the child looks up to him and perhaps enjoys activities with him that you don't. And they share genes, such that the son or daughter is a chip off the old block.

Some men don't struggle to see their wife as both mother and lover so much as they struggle to see themselves as both dad and lover. After all, a person only has so much time and energy. Such men may expect the lover to take a back seat while dad drives the car and keeps the family safe and well cared for.

But what about me? you say.

Yes, it's difficult to feel properly cared for when your relationship and sexual intimacy have been neglected. You want your children to have a fantastic dad, but you also want to have an attentive husband.

Change Begets Change

Charles Dickens wrote, "Change begets change. Nothing propagates so fast."[1] Propagating, a.k.a. reproducing, children may be the area where this is most true. You come home with something that weighs less than a gallon of paint, and suddenly your whole life has been recolored.

While "children are a gift of the LORD" (Ps. 127:3 NASB), they also strain many marriages. So many changes happen in this time that parents can struggle to find a new balance.

It's natural for parents to shift their focus to children. Caring for them is perhaps the most important thing we'll do in life. Yet we must also hold on to our oneness apart from the beautiful children we brought into the world. It's not selfish to do so. Children thrive in homes with the secure foundation of a mom and dad who are also friends and lovers.

So how can we keep love and passion alive? Well, we can't go back to the way it was before. Children equal change, and more changes come as they grow. Instead, we must embrace a new marriage-sustaining paradigm.

Making Space for Us

I wince every time some well-meaning person says to a group of couples, "Your marriage should always come before the children." Yes, strong families begin with solid marriages, so we should prioritize those relationships. But sometimes our kids should come before our marriage. Who wouldn't cancel a weekend away with their spouse if their child came down with pneumonia? Answer: bad parents.

Of course, that's a clear example. More often, we're faced with less obvious choices. How often should we go on a date night and leave our children with a babysitter? Should we take a family vacation or a romantic getaway? When should we allow our kid to interrupt our conversation or intimacy?

I don't have the answers for these questions, but too many couples fall into patterns without intentionality. They fail to talk about how to embrace their roles in an expanded family while continuing to make space for themselves as a couple. They don't discuss how their own views of each other have changed since becoming mom and dad, and where those views might need adjustment. They don't figure out a new way of relating sexually if or when the old way isn't working anymore.

To maintain a healthy sex life, you have to learn to shift from role to role—mom or dad to spouse/lover—and to carve out time for connection and passion. For the kinds of husbands I've described in this chapter, that's a challenging goal. But taking that first step or the next step, starting the conversation, or perhaps getting counseling can help the two of you make your way back to sex that works for both of you.

And it might produce another intrusive-but-remarkable child. Good luck with that!

CULTURAL INFLUENCES

I'm an American Gen Xer. My cohort is defined by growing up as latchkey kids, wearing neon colors and sporting big hair, watching Prince's *Purple Rain* movie, and expanding our screen options with cable and videotapes. We also remember the explosion of the *Challenger* shuttle, the Berlin Wall coming down, and the first video we saw on MTV, back when it was actually a music channel.

Of course, not everyone in my generation had the same experience. But our specific culture—including time, geography, events, technology, and influences—shapes us.

In this section, we'll address three issues that emanate from the culture that currently affects most of us and a fourth issue that's common in all cultures.

28. His Passivity

Before we discuss passivity, let's define it. Some hear a negative connotation with that word, but here's what "passive" means:

1. not reacting visibly to something that might be expected to produce manifestations of an emotion or feeling;
2. not participating readily or actively; inactive.[1]

Most of us have an area of life in which we're more passive than assertive, and that's fine. In this chapter, let's look at how a husband's passivity can impact his marriage's sexual intimacy.

From Labor to Leisure

After their wedding, my son and his wife moved into a cute little house in their college town and promptly settled into the joy of having their own place. Only the place didn't have a dishwasher. Having always lived in homes that did, they never thought to check for one. They were shocked to realize they had to wash their dishes the old-fashioned way—with soap, water, and elbow grease.

My mother would shake her head at that story.

My grandmother would laugh.

My great-grandmother would ask, "What's a dishwasher?"

Many of us live a less physically demanding life than our ancestors. We drive or ride in cars to our destinations. We cut our lawns with self-propelled lawn mowers. We order online and the purchase arrives at our doorstep.

In the last few centuries, many tasks have shifted from requiring manual labor to being performed with some automation. In recent decades, more tasks have shifted to computerization, and studies say the trend will continue. Moreover, tasks have moved inside—from laboring outdoors to completing work in warehouses, in stores, behind desks, and so on.

Why does any of this matter? Because it's taking a toll on men's collective sexual interest.

The Sedentary Life

While there's less physical risk involved in many jobs today, there's also less movement, less access to sunshine, and more stress. Each of these aspects can lead to a sexual desire deficit.

Exercise is imperative for good health. It doesn't have to be marathon running or mixed martial arts, but movement boosts our strength, heart health, energy, and testosterone. It used to be that people got enough movement in most jobs to keep things humming along okay. But that's not a given anymore. And if your husband spends a lot of time at his job, he may not have additional time in his schedule to get the exercise he needs to stay in shape.

Sunlight is also key for maintaining mood and sexual interest. Ultraviolet light increases testosterone, and a lack of it has the opposite effect. In addition, a vitamin D deficiency has been linked to lower testosterone and thus less sex drive. How do we get vitamin D? From three sources: food, supplements, and especially sunlight. In fact, it's sometimes called the "sunshine vitamin."[2] With a mostly indoors life, it's hard to get enough vitamin D.

Finally, stress has always been a part of work, but many men report feeling even more stressed in their current work environs.

Working long hours in cramped spaces without movement or sunshine can make us antsy, but add to that how we view the outcome. When a farmer sowed seed or a carpenter built houses or a railway worker laid tracks, they could see and touch the results of their labor. In the information and service economy, we have less tangible results. And that can lead to not feeling the same sense of reward.

Some men aren't well built for the sedentary life, and work and family pressures can make finding time for active endeavors difficult. Even if there is time, it can be more tempting to settle down and stream a show or play a video game. Those require less effort and are designed to make us feel a sense of accomplishment. Yet I'm convinced that all of us—and especially certain men—need opportunities and encouragement to take up work or hobbies that get us up and out and moving. They're good for our health, good for our mood, good for our mind, and, yes, good for our sex life.

Too Laid-Back to Get Laid

Speaking of leisure, some husbands are passive by personality. You may have been attracted to your man's easygoing approach to life, his ability to simply hang out and be in the moment, and the way life's stress passed over him like a wave.

But the flip side of a person's strength can be a weakness. What if that same attitude means he's not eager to expend energy on sex? For a more passive husband, it may feel like a lot of work to make sex happen, especially compared to all the other activities he or both of you could be doing.

Several wives have shared that their husband enjoys snuggling but doesn't seem that interested in sex, while other wives say that he might be interested but he's too laid-back to initiate.

When nothing else seems to be amiss, why aren't these men more eager to jump into such an enjoyable activity with their wife? Some of it may be the life of leisure we've grown accustomed to.

Also, there are many other possibilities for entertainment, and the laid-back husband may prefer feeling relaxed to feeling revved up.

Let's Get It Going

How can you address his sexual inactivity? Well, nagging at your husband to get off his bum and get to the bedroom has about a 0.05% chance of working, give or take 0.01%. So let's avoid that. Here are some better ways to help your husband get over the passivity hump.

Plan Together. Talk about how you could both spend free time better. Including yourself in the conversation makes it less of an accusation and more of a collaboration. Besides, we could all improve in that area, right? Then set *realistic* goals to become more active. Aiming too high and failing can shut down the desire to continue, but small gains can be built on. Some couples also introduce rewards; for example, walking the neighborhood together more days than not earns you two a dinner out.

Go Outside. Even if we're not doing anything active, sunlight and fresh air can perk us up. Your husband could take his laptop out to the patio table or play on his phone while lying in a hammock in the backyard. Or you could establish a "we time" on your front porch or apartment balcony where you spend a few minutes catching up over a cup of coffee, tea, or water. If you have kids, take them outside and sit nearby while they play.

Share a Project. Get your husband moving by suggesting something you can work on together. Maybe you've been wanting to paint a room, plant a garden, or build a compost bin. Make it a shared goal. If he says yes to the project but later balks about following through, remind him that most people struggle to begin and suggest he give it fifteen to twenty minutes and see if he gets into it. Oftentimes, once we start going, we're motivated to keep going.

Make the First Move. When it comes to sex, you're probably going to be the initiator for a while. Hopefully not the sole one, but the one with more rocket fuel to launch regular takeoffs. If this sounds unfair to you, you're right—and not. It's not fair for the responsibility of sexual intimacy to fall on you, yet marriage involves many times when one of you is better equipped for something and the other gets the benefit.

> Two are better than one,
>> because they have a good return for their labor:
> If either of them falls down,
>> one can help the other up.
> But pity anyone who falls
>> and has no one to help them up. (Eccles. 4:9–10)

In that scenario, the one standing pulls more weight than the one on the ground. Likewise, you may need to pull more weight in this area, while your husband lifts you up in other areas of your marriage.

So go ahead and initiate sex more than he does. You both might be glad if you do. He may want sex more often than he's admitted or even recognized, because it's a bigger challenge to him to get things going.

And strike while the iron is warm. Your passive husband may not ever heat up as much as you'd like, but he probably has certain days or times in the day when he's more active. Could you adjust your schedule for a sexual encounter then?

Finally, discuss with your husband ways that he might initiate sex that don't feel daunting to his more passive personality. You could come up with a secret phrase that connotes interest. I knew one couple who used "do taxes" as a euphemism for sex, though their children may have come away with a poor notion of how long it takes to file taxes. You could have visual signals, like a hand gesture or lighting a candle on the nightstand to indicate desire. There's always texting, with suggestive emojis or a word like "CHINA," which my colleague and good friend Chris

Taylor introduced me to as standing for "Come Home, I'm Naked Already."

Talk about what feels comfortable to him and how to navigate the challenges of his passivity. Sometimes understanding our husbands and meeting them where they are can create new ways of relating and getting things going in the bedroom as well.

29. Screen Time

Years back, my husband purchased a multilevel computer game that he played for hours each day. It frustrated me that he spent so much time with that game yet acted like a fifteen-minute conversation with me might kill him. (Don't worry—he survived.) I joked to friends that if he died and I was asked to identify his body, I'd request that the coroner flip him onto his stomach because I could better recognize the back of his head. After seeing the light himself, my husband deleted the game, and we've never had that problem again.

But it's a common one.

Many wives report losing their husband's attention, affection, and even sexual focus to TV, social media, video games, online news, and other activities on a screen. And getting those back can feel like wrestling a monitor-headed Godzilla to the ground.

Screen Time vs. Spouse Time

Most people underestimate their screen time. In a 2019 study of 2,000 baby boomers and millennials—as usual, skipping us Gen Xers—researchers concluded the average American spends 5.4 hours per day on their smartphone. Yet 82% of respondents thought their personal screen time was below the national average (impossible since, by definition, less than 50% can be below average).[1]

Today, the average American spends an estimated 7 hours 4 minutes looking at a screen every day.[2] Now, if you're like me and the vast majority of your job involves working on a computer, that doesn't seem so terrible. But 3 hours 40 minutes of that is social media or gaming, and some other portion is streaming TV or movies.[3] In other words, most of our screen time involves personal entertainment.

Meanwhile, how much time do we spend with our spouse?

That data is harder to come by, but the UK's Office for National Statistics suggested an average of 2.5 hours per day,[4] and a study published in the *Journal of Marriage and Family* in 2015 found that couples were exclusively together for about two hours on weekdays and three hours on weekends.[5] Since those match up pretty well, 2.5 hours seems to be a good estimate for couples generally.

Already, then, we spend an average of 1 hour 10 minutes more on screens than we do exclusively with our spouse. But wait, what about time couples spend watching a screen together? Shouldn't a husband get credit for that?

Men and women tend to view time spent together differently. According to researchers,

> Women report spending about 20 minutes less per day with their husbands than men report spending with their wives, even when diaries show agreement between husbands' and wives' activities. . . . This implies different interpretations of what counts as shared time as opposed to differences in actual time spent together. Evidence shows that husbands would like to have more time with their wives, but women would like more quality time with their husbands rather than simply more time together.[6]

What that means is that your husband might be counting that time you're sitting on the couch together engaged with a screen. But it might not feel like quality time to you.

Moreover, these are all averages, and your husband may spend far more time with screens than with you, inside or outside the bedroom.

How Screen Time Saps Sexual Interest

Some men spend several hours a day on screens and still have a strong sex drive. But for others, screen time decreases their sexual interest—often without them understanding what's going on. Let's consider why.

First, there's the issue of not enough time. With the regular demands of life, such as work, household duties, and parenting, plus sleep and screen time, how many hours are left to make love? Much less to romance, flirt, have foreplay, and enjoy afterglow? Not many.

A second major problem is dopamine. Dopamine is a neurotransmitter that sends messages between nerve cells, specifically ones that make us feel good. When we engage in an activity we find rewarding—eating a delicious meal, going shopping or dancing, or having great sex—our bodies release more dopamine, thus telling us to repeat the activity.

However, what happens on a screen often gives us a false sense of accomplishment, a virtual reward. Our bodies still get a dopamine rush that conveys, "You did it! Let's do it again." That's okay if our time on screens isn't excessive or involves focused work, but too much screen time teaches us to get dopamine hits without as much effort as real-world experiences—including sex, which takes intention, time, and effort.

Consider an intriguing study that reported gamers experience fewer problems with premature ejaculation than non-gamers.[7] Sounds great, right? Except:

Gamers reported lower levels of sexual satisfaction. . . . One explanation for lower rates of premature ejaculation could be due to gaming's ability to alter the brain's reward system.

In other words, men who play a lot of video games may be lasting longer in bed because they just aren't that into having sex.[8]

As one wife in my higher desire wife community stated, "Why put effort into relationships and sex that may take a little longer when you can get the same dopamine hit playing a game by yourself for less risk?"

Third, what a man sees on-screen can impact his view of sex. It doesn't have to be porn for your screen to show you something that isn't good for your sex life. Look up the most popular shows on Netflix and Amazon Prime, and you'll see that most of them are rated MA (mature audience), meaning they feature graphic violence, foul language, nudity, or some combination of the three. Video games feature voluptuous females built nothing like the average woman. Social media can also connect a husband with ex-girlfriends or show him eye candy.

The point is that the world sends constant messages about what women and sex should look like, and if husbands take large gulps of those messages, they can start expecting their wives or their sex life to look like the fictional version on-screen. When real life doesn't match those expectations, they may disengage.

Finally, while screen usage is not a sport, physical fatigue is a real thing. From eye strain and resultant headaches, to body aches from sitting in a particular pose or hunching over a keyboard or controller, to muscle tension and consequent exhaustion, a man can wear himself out. So much so that a tumble in the sheets could feel like a draw on his last reserves.

Trading One Joystick for Another

Your husband may spend so much time with his game controller's joystick that you don't get to spend enough time with his joystick. How can you get him to understand the negative impact screen time is having on your sexual intimacy and marriage?

188

Before you announce that his screen obsession is ruining your sex life—a tactic unlikely to yield a good result—start with a more basic question: how often are we on screens? Yes, *we*. Remember that most of us underestimate our screen time. Suggest to your husband that you each guess how much time you spend on your phone, tablet, TV, desktop, laptop, gaming console, etc., and then track it over a week or two. Report back and talk through how well you did with your guesses and what you think of the reality. You may find that your own usage needs adjustment, and that's both a good place to start and an example for him.

Hopefully, he'll want to make adjustments too. If so, you can support one another with encouragement, accountability, and external rewards to maintain progress. You could suggest dinner out or another dopamine-hit activity if you get your screen hours down to a certain level.

If he's resistant, talk about what you're seeing in your relationship, why you're concerned about his screen use, and how much you miss him. If he's willing, you might suggest he try X number of hours fewer one week and see how things go. A successful trial run might free him from the dopamine rushes long enough to better grasp what's been happening.

But if he seems to be in the black hole of screen addiction—spending numerous hours, acting irritated and defensive, being unwilling to try something different—you may want to speak to a trusted loved one in his life. Perhaps a best friend or mentor can get through where you can't, especially if they've witnessed his inability to step away.

If or when you can get your husband away from the TV remote, computer mouse, or game controller, it may take time to rebuild sexual interest and intimacy. His nervous system needs to reconfigure the dopamine hits to come after more effort and in response to real-life stimuli. Remind your husband that's just the process and the destination is worth the journey.

30. Forbidden Fruit

Elizabeth is happily married to her second husband, her first marriage having rightfully gone the way of the dodo. In addition to enduring abuse from her ex-husband, she was shut out sexually. Their physical intimacy started during their engagement, but as she described it, something odd happened right after the "I dos."

> When we thought that we were in love and were going to get married, that's when we started up a sexual relationship. And at that time, it was like, *I can't keep my hands off of you.* And it was very passionate.
>
> We got married, and on our wedding night, I was the initiator, and so we did have sex on our wedding night. The second night that we were married, I put on something that I hoped would make me look appealing and be appealing, and it was, "Oh no, I'm not in the mood for that right now." Our honeymoon ended up being a week long, and I tried every night and we never made love for the whole trip.

For the remainder of their marriage, her husband rejected sexual intimacy again and again. Comparing before the wedding to after, Elizabeth said, "It was like it changed on a dime."

She isn't alone. I've heard similar stories multiple times:

- "He had a really hard time stopping before we got married, but now he isn't interested."

- "We made love once and it was amazing, but then we decided to wait until our wedding night. I wish we hadn't because he didn't want to once we got married."
- "Based on how we made out, I was sure we were going to have a great sex life. But now that we're married . . ."

Women who find themselves in a similar situation often wonder, *What happened to the man who was eager to have sex before marriage? Did slipping on the wedding ring cut off the circulation of his sex drive?*

Danger Zone

"Psychological reactance" refers to how telling someone they can't have or do something often results in them experiencing greater desire to have or do that thing.

We tend to test boundaries, push the envelope, see what might be behind that closed door or sealed box. (Stop peeking, Pandora!) Let's say you know you shouldn't get into the cookie jar before dinner, and you open it one night to find . . . roaches. If you're anything like me, you'll slam that lid closed and wait for supper. However, if you open up the cookie jar and find delicious cookies, you might have one. Or two. You might even get in the habit of sneaking a cookie or two now and then.

For a lot of folks, that describes sex. They were told so often that they shouldn't have sex before marriage that some part of them reared up and said, "Hey, don't tell me what to do!" Or they were at least curious about what they were being kept from. So they took a taste and found it wasn't roaches but a really good cookie. They even felt a hit of dopamine, a neurochemical that serves as a satisfying reward to the system.

Very quickly, the motivation became not the cookie itself or not the cookie alone. Rather, it was as much or more about being in the danger zone—bucking rules, exerting personal freedom, experiencing psychological reactance.

Adam and Eve

We learn about the first partakers of a forbidden fruit way back in Genesis. God tells Adam and Eve, "Enjoy all these things in the garden! Oh, except that one tree. Don't eat from it, and things will be fine" (paraphrased, of course). And what did they do? They ate the fruit from the one tree they weren't supposed to have.

Shame came later, but while they were eating? "When the woman saw that the fruit of the tree was good for food and pleasing to the eye, and also desirable for gaining wisdom, she took some and ate it. She also gave some to her husband, who was with her, and he ate it" (Gen. 3:6). They enjoyed it in the moment.

Thankfully, God cut them off from that tree and its fruit. Otherwise, they might have had the experience some Christians have with sex—knowing they shouldn't have sex before marriage but doing it anyway and discovering that not only is it a yummy fruit, there's an adrenaline rush from tasting forbidden fruit. Even if they felt shame afterward, they return to that fruit again and again. Over time, shame fades and that adrenaline rush becomes an integral part of what makes sex feel good.

What happens when a man with this experience etched into his memory and feelings gets married? He might get through the wedding night or honeymoon, but sex soon loses its appeal because it's not taboo anymore. Without forbidden fruit, sex simply doesn't arouse or satisfy.

Now Wed, Is Sex Dead?

Some husbands respond by attempting to introduce forbidden fruit into the marriage relationship—rough lovemaking, fringe activities, or dangerous scenarios, such as having sex in a public place where they could get caught.

Other husbands turn to forbidden fruit outside the marriage—pornography, paid sexual encounters (for example, lap dances or prostitution), or adultery. Having realized that sex approved by God and society isn't doing it for them, they seek arousal and satisfaction elsewhere.

Yet other husbands retreat from marital sex altogether, because it's just not firing their cylinders. A lower desire husband in this situation may not understand why sex no longer interests him. Or he might know why he's not interested, specifically because sex no longer feels like living on the edge, and he doesn't want to suggest danger-zone activities to his wife simply to get his engine revving like it did before. Forbidden fruit is what his habit-formed mind and body want, but his conscience won't let him go there.

In the first scenario—a man subjecting his wife to forbidden fruit options—the husband devalues intimacy with his wife. Women in such circumstances have emailed me through the years, and they justifiably feel pressured, used, and unsafe.

In the other two scenarios—a man who turns elsewhere and a man who retreats—the husband disengages from intimacy with his wife. Although the result is the same—a rejected wife—these are obviously different perspectives that require different responses. So let's take these three scenarios in turn.

An Immoral Husband

Aria's husband isn't as low drive as their sexual frequency would indicate. He'd engage in sex more *if* she'd do the things he wants. But what he wants shows far less interest in intimacy than forbidden fruit. As Aria explained, "What he wants oftentimes crosses boundaries that I convictionally believe are not okay."

Aria went on to tell me some of her husband's specific requests: watching pornography together, her having sex with other men while he watches, and others watching the two of them have sex.

While he might claim he's available for sex more often, he's really not. He's interested in sexual sin rather than connection with his wife. His desire for true sexual intimacy is very low, leaving Aria feeling rejected and deprived of what God intends their marriage to have.

A wife shouldn't cooperate with sin! Scripture makes it clear that we can defy even authorities we should otherwise submit to when they suggest sin, but our husband isn't the authority regarding our sexual intimacy. He's a mutual partner in the bedroom, and God calls him to love his wife "as Christ loved the church and gave himself up for her to make her holy, cleansing her by the washing with water through the word, and to present her to himself as a radiant church, without stain or wrinkle or any other blemish, but holy and blameless" (Eph. 5:25–27).

Even though it's left Aria without the sex she longs to have with her husband, she made the correct choice by refusing to engage in his unholy fantasies. She's holding out for the intimacy her marriage deserves.

An Unfaithful Husband

We've already addressed some examples of unfaithfulness (see chapters 22–24). But the pull of forbidden fruit can also lead some husbands to infidelity.

Remember Elizabeth, the wife at the beginning of this chapter whose first husband disengaged right after the wedding night? Over the years, she learned that he viewed a lot of pornography, engaged in online sex chats, and had one-night stands. All while turning down her sexual advances and pleas for intimacy. For that marriage to have a shot at surviving, he needed a change of heart. Sadly, he didn't get there, but many other men have.

Some husbands make no excuses about what they're doing, perhaps even flaunting their behavior, but most hide from their wife and others, living a double life. John 3:20 says, "All who do evil hate the light and refuse to go near it for fear their sins will be

194

exposed" (NLT). But only by bringing their sinful behavior into the light can it be faced and fixed. That might involve you asking questions, giving greater thought to red flags you've noticed, or confronting him.

Please don't lob accusations with no evidence. If he's not being unfaithful and you accuse him of infidelity, then you've introduced a fresh obstacle to physical intimacy—an unwarranted lack of trust. But if you have confirmation, you should bring what you know to light because it needs to be dealt with. Consider what else Scripture has to say on this matter:

> Take no part in the worthless deeds of evil and darkness; instead, expose them. It is shameful even to talk about the things that ungodly people do in secret. But their evil intentions will be exposed when the light shines on them, for the light makes everything visible. (Eph. 5:11–14 NLT)

Take no part in your husband's "worthless deeds," but rather help him find the light. Bringing sin out into the open is only the first step, but it's an important one.

Throughout this process, feel free to own your hurt, express your anger, and grieve the loss of trust in your marriage. You can share some of what you feel with your husband, who needs to understand the impact of his actions. Not in a way that you sin as well, but giving voice to appropriate emotions. Feel free to unload when you're alone, in the pages of your personal journal, in a session with your therapist, and definitely with God. For guidance, read through the psalms of lament, such as Psalms 3, 13, 22, 42, and 86. These poems express sorrow, petition God for help, and often end with a glimpse of hope.

An Avoidant Husband

A husband who avoids sex altogether blocks both himself and his wife from physical intimacy. While it's good that he's avoiding the temptation to take bites of forbidden fruit, he's also missing out on all the good fruit God gave a thumbs-up to—specifically, satisfying sexual experiences with a loving wife.

The problem is that he doesn't know that non-forbidden fruit can taste great *and* be truly satisfying. He has to be convinced, and that requires time and effort to rewrite the scripts.

Think about it like sugar. For most of my life, I loved sugar—from glazed donuts to Coca-Cola to rich desserts. I knew I should eat more fruits, but fruit-flavored items (with generous amounts of sugar) tasted so much better.

In May 2023, however, I discovered the root of a constellation of symptoms I was experiencing: body aches, headaches, joint pain, fatigue, heartburn, and heart palpitations. I had food sensitivities, including an extreme reaction to sugar. Within a few weeks, I became completely sugar free. And weirdly, wonderfully, I came to realize how delicious fruit really is! No longer was it something I had to remind myself to eat. Instead, eating a bowl of fruit felt like indulging in a sweet treat.

Suggest to your avoidant husband that, as a couple, you relearn how to make love in a way that works for both of you. Acknowledge that it won't be the way he thought it would be, but you want to take time to create something healthy and satisfying for both of you. Ask him to give it time, and expect to take it slow.

If possible, schedule sex for a while, to make sure you have enough encounters to begin rewriting the script stuck in his head. Weekly is a good place to start, and you can choose a day of the week to put on the calendar or a time period such as the weekend.

Over time, the scales can shift, and the bulk of his sexual experiences will be positive, real ones within the sacred space of marriage. And he'll discover that this fruit is a sweeter treat than anything he knew before.

31. Just Mismatched

For fifteen years, Babette searched for an answer to why her husband's drive was lower than hers. She asked many of the same questions you've likely asked yourself and explored some possibilities we've covered. In the end, she concluded,

> I don't think it's anything physical. I don't think— It's not pornography. It's nothing like that. I just think we have a different sex drive. I told him if I had married someone else, then I may have been the lesser drive spouse and the same with him. He could have been the higher drive. I think it's just a ratio.

Babette put words to a dynamic we touched on in an earlier chapter: "higher drive" and "lower drive" are relative terms. Sometimes a mismatch in sex drives doesn't indicate a problem. Rather, it's how one husband and one wife happen to fall on the spectrum of sexual desire.

In a guest post on my site, titled "Sexual Desire Differences: What If There's Nothing Going Wrong?," Dr. Corey Allan, marriage therapist and host of *Sexy Marriage Radio*, put it this way:

> There's always a low desire spouse and there's always a high desire spouse—and there's one of each in every marriage.
>
> There's a low desire spouse and a high desire spouse on virtually every issue and decision in marriage. One of you wants to do something the other doesn't, or wants to less than you. And even

if you both want the same thing, one of you will want it more than the other. Plus, no one is the low desire, or high desire on everything. Positions shift on different issues throughout the marriage.[1]

While there may be a good reason why your husband doesn't want sex as much as you do—thus the long list of options in this book—it's also possible that it's a simple mismatch. Even if both of you had a perfect relationship otherwise, you'd still come out as the higher desire spouse.

God intended sexual intimacy to be *mutually* desired and enjoyed, but just like conversation and affection, it doesn't have to be *equally* desired and enjoyed. Your husband may want and value sex, just not as much as you do. If that's your story, that's okey-dokey.

You can still have a fulfilling marriage that includes sexual intimacy. You may need to tweak your expectations and your approach, but you can enjoy a wonderful sexual intimacy together, appreciating how God made you to fit together according to his design.

PART 3

WHY IS YOUR DRIVE HIGHER?

So far, we've looked at a number of reasons why your husband's sexual interest may be lower. But it's also worth asking why yours is higher.

Why is your libido where it is? And what does it say about you?

32. What's Healthy and Holy?

While the first message I want to get out to higher desire wives is "you're not alone," the second is "there's nothing wrong with a wife being the higher desire spouse."

After covering so many issues that could be keeping your husband from desiring or enjoying sex as much as you do, we also need to spend some time talking about whether your specific experience of a higher sex drive is healthy and holy. Some women take sex out of its rightful context as an important type of marital intimacy and elevate it to an idol or use it as a balm to soothe broken places inside them. Understandable, but not ideal.

What Does Sex Mean to You?

I encourage spouses to ask one another this question and to dig deep with their answers. Here's a sampling of responses I've heard from wives:

- "Sex is a husband's need that I meet because Scripture tells me to."
- "Sex means ceding control of my body, and I hate that because I was abused as a child."
- "Sex means I'm desirable and loved."

- "Sex is the way to get children but doesn't mean much else to me."
- "Sex is something I need and deserve."

You might not relate to any of those answers. Instead, you might say something like, "Sex is a physical way to express and nurture the love and commitment I have with my husband." And I'd high-five you for an answer like that! But is that all sex means to you?

Dig deep. Do you measure your worth in some way by your sex life? Do you feel like God owes you the fantastic sex everyone talked about because you waited until your wedding night? Did your past use of pornography or erotica create unreasonable expectations that focus more on pleasure than intimacy? Did past abuse or mistreatment make you determined to be in control—to have sex on your own terms? Did an unhealthy relationship with your father make you more needy of male affection and reassurance than you otherwise would be?

These are tough questions, and the answers may summon negative feelings. But it's worth asking how we've framed sexuality for ourselves and whether we need to adjust our views to fall better within God's design.

Sex Soothes, but It Doesn't Heal

I grew up before the purity culture of the 1990s to 2000s, but the message of "DON'T" was conveyed very clearly. Don't have sex, don't want sex, don't think about sex—until you get married. But, as you read earlier, I couldn't not think about sex. My body reminded me all too often that I was drawn to guys, experienced odd physical sensations around them, and wondered what other sensations might be available. I was, as God made me, a sexual being.

In addition to that, I had daddy issues. I know that's a cliché, but there's truth to it. Some women crave physical attention from a man because they didn't receive it from a loving father. My father had a severe temper, and after a while, I no longer wanted him to hug or be close to me. I simply couldn't reconcile his mistreatment with affection. But that left a hole in my life that needed filling. One way to get the male touch I wanted was to make myself more available to guys.

Given that bone-deep craving for male affection, and figuring I'd already crossed into sin territory by often thinking about and wanting sex, I fell into premarital promiscuity. I won't lie—the physical sensations were enjoyable, and the ache for attention eased. But such moments were fleeting and left me once again feeling empty. Or emptier than before. The whole experience broke my heart, wounded others, and fractured my relationship with God.

I needed healing, but I sought soothing. Sex could soothe, but it couldn't heal.

What I experienced before marriage is true within marriage as well. Many of us look to sex to soothe our wounds, fill our gaps, affirm our identities, and sate our hunger—yet we end up emptier and hungrier than before. Because what we need is healing.

My healing included diving into Scripture to discover what God really says about sex, using cognitive-behavioral techniques and Scripture meditations to embrace that new paradigm, and personal counseling. You might find a similar path to be helpful, or you may take a different path. As I've said before, if your past involves abuse, addiction, or adultery, please see a professional counselor. But even if you haven't experienced those, you might benefit from therapy.

Whether you pursue therapy or not, many resources can help you move toward healing, such as those named in other chapters. At the top of the list is our handy-dandy guide to life, the Bible.

What's a Healthy, Holy Sex Drive?

Identifying the factors that have influenced your thoughts and feelings about sex is a great place to start. But it's not enough to know where things have gone awry. You need to know what you're aiming for. How do you know if your sex drive is in line with God's design? Is your stronger desire for sexual intimacy healthy and holy?

First, how often do you feel that you need to have sex? Not long ago, a wife sent me an email explaining her husband expected sex at least daily and got upset when he didn't get it. I responded that that's not normal. While daily sex sounds pretty good to me, a spouse should be able to go without for a few days without becoming distressed.

When I asked my higher desire community, "How long can you go without sex before you start to feel antsy?" the number one answer was three to four days, with the number two answer being five to seven days. That's consistent with a healthy frequency, with research showing that one to two times per week sufficiently nurtures marital intimacy.[1]

If you feel jittery or upset if you don't have sex nearly every day, you may need to ask whether your expectations are reasonable. Healthy sexual intimacy in marriage doesn't mean getting sex every single time you want it, but rather coming up with an amount that's both good for the marriage and satisfactory for each spouse.

Second, how much of your identity is wrapped up in your sexuality? Let's look at my life as an example. In addition to my daddy issues and the "just don't" message I received while growing up, I wasn't a pretty girl. I was awkward and too skinny and a VIP member of the Itty Bitty Titty Club. Once I became sexually active, a large part of feeling better about my appearance relied on being sexually desired.

You may measure your own appearance or worth by your sexuality. Now, it's understandable to question your attractiveness when your husband isn't interested in sex with you. But stretch your mind back to before marriage or even before meeting your husband. What did you anticipate being sexual would say about you? Would it mean you were beautiful? Important? Powerful?

Fully woman? Or consider how you felt when you first had sex. Did you feel it made you more whole than you were before?

Sex in marriage does say something about you—hopefully, that you're in a covenant marriage and committed to expressing and nurturing intimacy with your husband. But it's nowhere near the most important thing about you. It doesn't make you more worthy in some way. If tomorrow you were entirely incapable of having sex, you'd still be just as beautiful, important, and womanly as before. You'd still be God's precious daughter.

It's healthy to believe what God says about who we are and bring that whole person into the marriage bed to join with another. Can we reach that level of wholeness, of feeling confidently lovable and loved? Maybe not 100%, but if we let sex define us, we've got the wrong dictionary. We need to replace the erroneous messages we're telling ourselves with higher truth.

Which brings us back to the Bible showing us the way to heal. Take some time to meditate on the following passage. Read it daily, memorize it, and remind yourself that this—not any aspect of your sexuality or your sex life—is God's true measure for your worth.

> For you created my inmost being;
> you knit me together in my mother's womb.
> I praise you because I am fearfully and wonderfully made;
> your works are wonderful,
> I know that full well. (Ps. 139:13–14)

Third, how do you react to a "no"? I constantly coach lower desire spouses to avoid saying "no" and to instead say "not now" (along with when might be a better time) when they aren't interested in having sex. But they aren't the only ones who can defuse the tension of competing desire levels. We higher desire spouses have an obligation to respond appropriately to being turned down.

When your husband doesn't catch your hints, doesn't respond to your advances, or outright rejects an offer of sex, do you express disappointment but move on? Or do you show frustration and anger? Pout or cry? Distance yourself as punishment?

If it's been a long time, you may experience emotional pain. By now, I hope you understand that I get it—how hurtful it can be to desire your husband so much and feel that he doesn't have the same longing for you.

But I also hope you've seen that he's likely not thinking of sex in those terms. Any number of reasons, which have little to nothing to do with you, could cause him to say no to a sexual encounter. So while you can and should lean into your grief, take it to God and find friends and resources to help you address it. There's a good way and a bad way to respond to your husband's lower sexual interest. If his no creates a storm in you that leads you to lash out at him, he's less likely to say yes the next time.

And you should ask why the storm rages so strong. Are your reactions in proportion to what's happening, or does his rejection tap into another deep hurt that hasn't healed? One way to think through this possibility is to ask, *When else in my life have I felt this way?* Do your feelings resemble moments from your past when you felt abandoned or unwanted? Maybe by a parent or in a prior relationship?

Your answers to these questions may tell you that it's time to seek that deeper healing through prayer, meditation on God's Word, therapy, a support group, or something else. That doesn't mean your sex life shouldn't improve. But pursuing healing means putting sex into its proper place and not expecting it to do what it cannot do.

Feeding the Wrong Wolf

Perhaps you've heard the parable of the two wolves. A grandfather explains to his grandson that the conflict between good and bad is like two wolves wrestling. When his grandson asks which wolf will win, the grandfather replies, "Whichever one you feed."

Sexual desire and intimacy as God intended is the good wolf, but if twisted, sex can become the bad wolf.

All too often, we're feeding the wrong wolf. We think we're pursuing sex as intimacy with our husband, but we're really seeking it out for other reasons—often to plug an emptiness inside us that sex can't fill.

Are you feeding your mind expectations your husband cannot live up to through what you read, watch, fantasize about, and compare your husband to? Do you focus on sexual intimacy to the exclusion of other forms of intimacy in your marriage? Do you measure your marriage or worth based on how the sex is going? Do you dwell on hurt and resentment, stirring them up until they're nearly foaming over?

What about the good wolf? Do you meditate on Scriptures that remind you of your worth and God's love? Do you look at your husband not just with frustration but also with compassion? Do you seek out ways to be intimate that aren't sexual? Do you encourage teamwork in addressing sexual gaps in your marriage? Do you exhibit the fruit of the Spirit as you seek more satisfying sex with your husband?

We higher desire wives can feed the wrong wolf and then wonder why we feel so chewed up. Mind you, the good-wolf route isn't pain free. But whatever's happening with our sex life and our husband, we have the power and responsibility to choose healthy and holy sexuality for ourselves.

We can put sex in its proper place—as a good gift from God that shows and grows intimacy in marriage but doesn't define us or our relationship and cannot heal our broken places. That job belongs to Christ.

33. Higher Desire Wives in the Bible

Do you have a favorite Bible character? Mine is the apostle Peter. I relate to how he failed so many times but kept getting back up and trying again, until finally he became the hero of faith he wanted to be. I'm not yet the hero of faith I want to be! But I find comfort in knowing that we can mess up multiple times, repent and receive God's grace, and start over with the slate wiped clean.

Perhaps your favorite person from the Bible is someone you relate to as well. But what about being a higher desire wife? Is there anyone in Scripture you can relate to? Anyone who gets it and gives you hope?

Higher desire wives are not a new phenomenon. They've always existed, including wives from biblical times. Let's talk about these wives and how their sexual desire was perceived, starting with the surprising Judaic view of a woman's sexuality.

The Mitzvah of Onah

Christianity is the fulfillment of Judaic law, meaning that Jesus's coming was not a brand-new thing that erased prior history but rather the perfection of God's plan all along. Accordingly, we can learn a lot from the Old Testament about who God is and what he wants, even if certain commands no longer apply.

With that in mind, let's look at Exodus 21:10: "If [a man] takes an additional wife, he must not reduce the food, clothing, or marital rights of the first wife" (HCSB).

Maybe you're bothered by that phrase "additional wife." So am I. Polygamy was never God's intent, but it had become part of the Israelites' culture, and God's response was to do what was possible in that context to protect women. Rather than going off on that tangent, let's consider God's heart for wives during those times. If a man planned to take a second wife, he was instructed not to reduce what the first wife was getting, including her "marital rights." Other translations replace that phrase with "conjugal rights" or even "sexual intimacy."

Based on this one verse and the intent behind it, Jewish priests and scholars developed broader explanations for husbands regarding this duty. It's called the mitzvah (command) of onah (time of lovemaking), and it has come to mean this:

> Sex is the woman's right, not the man's. A man has a duty to give his wife sex regularly and to ensure that sex is pleasurable for her. He is also obligated to watch for signs that his wife wants sex, and to offer it to her without her asking for it.[1]

The idea of sex as the woman's right is foreign to many today, yet it wasn't such a crazy notion then. In fact, another verse sheds light on the expectation that wives wanted and deserved to have sex in marriage:

> If a man has recently married, he must not be sent to war or have any other duty laid on him. For one year he is to be free to stay at home and bring happiness to the wife he has married. (Deut. 24:5)

While "bring happiness" doesn't equal "have sex," Israelites understood that the first year was a time for the couple to establish a home, learn how to love one another, and experience sexual intimacy. And the command is given to the husband to keep his wife happy.

Does that mean husbands owe their wives joyful sexual intimacy but wives don't owe their husbands the same in return? While the word "owe" comes with baggage I don't want to give it, many other places in Scripture make it clear that God intends for both spouses to prioritize sexual intimacy.

Someone may ask, "Isn't this verse just about having kids?" Perhaps this command reflects the commandment to Adam and Eve to "be fruitful and multiply" (Gen. 1:28 NKJV)? Except that's not how the verse is typically interpreted by theologians. Children might come from sexual intimacy between a husband and wife, but they're not the only goal, or the commands would not talk about marital rights or a wife's happiness but rather producing children.

God gave women sexual desire and then honored that gift by encouraging men to meet their longing for physical intimacy in the rightful context of marriage. Booyah! Right?

Now let's move on to specific higher desire wives in the Bible.

Potiphar's Wife

The first woman I can easily identify as having strong sexual desire was not a biblical heroine. Potiphar's wife was an Egyptian adulteress whose lies about Joseph landed him in jail for years. Hardly the role model we want! But while I'd never condone her awful behavior, it's interesting how passionately she sought out sex with Joseph. What was going on with her?

Potiphar purchased Joseph as a slave and eventually "put him in charge of his household, and he entrusted to his care everything he owned" (Gen. 39:4). While the story doesn't say that Potiphar was often gone, his job was captain of Pharaoh's guard, a military position that likely involved travel—to conquer others and all that jazz. Given what we read about the mitzvah of onah, it's reasonable to wonder: Did she get her year of happiness in their first year of marriage? Or was she expected to be there when he was ready, but not sure what value she had otherwise? We don't know.

What we do know is that Potiphar's wife wanted sex and was willing to initiate it with a young man not her husband. "Now Joseph was well-built and handsome, and after a while his master's wife took notice of Joseph and said, 'Come to bed with me!'" (vv. 6–7).

She was also persistent. "Though she spoke to Joseph day after day, he refused to go to bed with her or even be with her" (Gen. 39:10).

She's *not* our hero, but can you relate to the desire? I can.

And Scripture doesn't say that her longing for sexual intimacy was bad. Had this story been about a woman initiating sex with her husband, and perhaps even his refusal, how do you think Scripture would have recorded it? Would her desires in those circumstances have been against God? Of course not.

While we might say to ourselves, "But that's not me! I'd never do that," let me share what many higher desire wives have told me. When a woman doesn't get the sexual intimacy she wants from her husband, especially if the refusal continues for a long time, she can become vulnerable to the temptation of an affair.

We can feel some affinity with Potiphar's wife's desire for sex, but we'd be wise to take her story as a warning. Let's make sure our desires are directed where they belong—toward our husband.

Bathsheba (Maybe)

Asked about the most controversial people in the Bible, I'd put Bathsheba high on the list. Some have seen Bathsheba as a temptress bathing on her roof where the overwhelmed king could see her. Some have seen her as a victim targeted and raped by a predatory king. And many explanations rest in between these interpretations. While I have my own theory, I don't want to talk about Bathsheba's relationship with David but rather her relationship with her first husband, Uriah the Hittite.

Uriah was one of David's mighty warriors, men who fought valiantly for and alongside the king. He was a military man who spent a fair amount of time away from home, especially "in the spring, at the time when kings go off to war" (2 Sam. 11:1). After whatever happened between her and David, Bathsheba turned up pregnant. King David summoned Uriah and encouraged him to go home and spend time with his wife, wanting to hide his own infidelity with Bathsheba. But Uriah didn't know that at the time. Here's how the exchange is recorded:

> David said to Uriah, "Go down to your house and wash your feet." So Uriah left the palace, and a gift from the king was sent after him. But Uriah slept at the entrance to the palace with all his master's servants and did not go down to his house.
>
> David was told, "Uriah did not go home." So he asked Uriah, "Haven't you just come from a military campaign? Why didn't you go home?"
>
> Uriah said to David, "The ark and Israel and Judah are staying in tents, and my commander Joab and my lord's men are camped in the open country. How could I go to my house to eat and drink and make love to my wife? As surely as you live, I will not do such a thing!" (2 Sam. 11:8–11)

My Bible teachers always cast Uriah's actions as honorable and selfless, and yes, that's a reasonable interpretation. But from the wife's perspective, how would you feel about this? Your husband, who may die in war and has been gone for a long time, passes up the opportunity to be physically intimate with you and thus reassure you of his love. Does anything about that sound familiar?

Again, I have no idea how Bathsheba felt about Uriah and that decision or about David—though he clearly took advantage of his position in securing her—but if she wanted her husband's sexual attention, she didn't get it. That rejection and the longing left in its wake is something many of us can relate to.

The Shulammite Woman

Song of Songs is a collection of love poetry involving a married couple who speak of romantic and sexual desire for one another. It begins with the woman saying,

> Let him kiss me with the kisses of his mouth—
>   for your love is more delightful than wine.
> Pleasing is the fragrance of your perfumes;
>   your name is like perfume poured out.
>   No wonder the young women love you!
> Take me away with you—let us hurry!
>   Let the king bring me into his chambers. (1:2–4)

That sounds like a woman rarin' to go!

It would appear that she and her beloved husband are well matched in sexual interest. Their back-and-forth exchanges indicate that they both desire and appreciate sexual intimacy. Even if she has a high sex drive, we can't say that it's higher than her husband's.

I don't contend that the Shulammite woman (as she's identified in 6:13) wants sex more in their marriage. What I do see is that they each experience wanting sex and being left hanging.

> I slept but my heart was awake.
>   Listen! My beloved is knocking:
> "Open to me, my sister, my darling,
>   my dove, my flawless one.
> My head is drenched with dew,
>   my hair with the dampness of the night."
> I have taken off my robe—
>   must I put it on again?

> I have washed my feet—
>   must I soil them again? (5:2–3)

Her husband initiates, and what's her response? It's late, she's tired, and she doesn't want to get up and answer the door, even for sex. But then:

> My beloved thrust his hand through the latch-opening;
>   my heart began to pound for him.
> I arose to open for my beloved,
>   and my hands dripped with myrrh,
> my fingers with flowing myrrh,
>   on the handles of the bolt.
> I opened for my beloved,
>   but my beloved had left; he was gone.
>   My heart sank at his departure.
> I looked for him but did not find him.
>   I called him but he did not answer. . . .
> Daughters of Jerusalem, I charge you—
>   if you find my beloved,
> what will you tell him?
>   Tell him I am faint with love. (vv. 4–6, 8)

Now she wants sex, but he's nowhere to be found.

In the book, these experiences come one right after the other, though Song of Songs is not a linear story but rather a poetic telling of romantic desire and sexual intimacy in marriage. These verses, then, can be seen to represent a season in a marriage, and many higher desire wives can relate to that latter passage.

Perhaps you weren't always the higher desire spouse. Rather, he was once more interested than you or you were well matched, but now when you want sex, your husband's nowhere to be found. What happened? Doesn't he see that you are "faint with love"?

214

The Song of Songs wife felt that heart-sinking disappointment of desiring sexual intimacy with her husband, calling for him, and not getting an answer. She knows.

Corinthian Widows

If 1 Corinthians 13 is the love chapter, then 1 Corinthians 7 is the sex chapter. It begins with "now for the matters you wrote about" (v. 1), meaning Paul is addressing questions posed by the church at Corinth.

In particular, it seems some Corinthians had concluded that if sex outside of marriage—including temple prostitution—was off-limits, maybe all sex was less-than. Wouldn't it be better to devote oneself to spiritual activities and avoid physical ones? Isn't sex an ungodly experience, even if it's necessary for children? That conclusion isn't too far removed from what many throughout church history have believed—that sex was not approved by God except to meet his command to be fruitful and multiply. However, Paul's answer reaffirms that God planned for sex to be a part of marriage, whether or not it produces children. (Indeed, the one mention of children in 1 Corinthians 7 has nothing to do with sex but with staying married to an unbeliever.)

One way that Paul affirmed God's view of sex was in his counsel regarding Corinthian widows: "I say to the unmarried and to widows: It is good for them if they remain as I am. But if they do not have self-control, they should marry, for it is better to marry than to burn with desire" (1 Cor. 7:8–9 HCSB).

Remember that Paul is living at a time when persecution is amping up and believers think time is very limited. As much as they got right about Christ, they couldn't have imagined having brothers and sisters of the faith living in the twenty-first century. In that context, it makes a lot of sense for Paul to suggest it would be "good for them if they remain as I am" as they await the imminent return of Christ.

Yet Paul expects that some singles—including widows, who'd experienced physical intimacy with a husband—would struggle mightily to go without sex. One could ding them as not having sufficient self-control, but Paul doesn't say they are lesser Christians. He says to go ahead, get married, and, yes, have sex.

Why would he say that if he didn't recognize that plenty of women have a strong sex drive? As high or higher than some men?

If I could time travel to first-century Corinth, it wouldn't take long for me to come across one of these widows, recline at a table with bread and wine, and share how much we enjoyed sexual intimacy with our husbands. And some of those wives would marry again, because they desire both marriage and the sex God intended them to have within it.

Equal Opportunity Desire

While the Jewish orthodox view of sex is that it's a wife's right, much of Scripture, including Song of Songs and 1 Corinthians 7, indicates that sex can and should be desired by both husbands and wives.

> The husband should fulfill his marital duty to his wife, and likewise the wife to her husband. The wife does not have authority over her own body but yields it to her husband. In the same way, the husband does not have authority over his own body but yields it to his wife. Do not deprive each other except perhaps by mutual consent and for a time, so that you may devote yourselves to prayer. Then come together again so that Satan will not tempt you because of your lack of self-control. (1 Cor. 7:3–5)

If you've ever heard a lesson or sermon on this verse, you probably heard an emphasis on wives needing to meet a husband's sexual needs. But that's not what this passage says.

Rather, it addresses the reality that some Corinthians were withholding sex in marriage, believing it was godlier to avoid sex altogether. Paul reassures husbands and wives that sex is an important component of marriage—even a "duty." He paints the picture of a husband and wife yielding to one another and coming together regularly.

And he does all that by starting not with the husband's needs but with the wife's: "The husband should fulfill his marital duty to his wife" (v. 3). *She* is owed sex.

As soon as I wrote that, I panicked. Because I know how someone could pull my words out of context, saying that I'm telling lower desire spouses they have a duty to have sex even when they don't want it, or I'm telling higher desire spouses they can demand the sex they're owed. I'm *not* saying that!

Just because we have a duty to do something doesn't mean we have to do it today or when we have reasons to resist. Nor does our spouse owing us something mean we can ever use force, demands, or pressure to get it. As my good friend and podcast cohost, Gaye Christmus, often says, "Christianity is never about demanding your rights."

Paul's message here is that God planned for sex to be a part of marriage, and he expected that both wives and husbands would want and enjoy this gift. The higher desire women of the Bible and in our time are not anomalies but exactly what God anticipated.

So why is your sex drive higher than your husband's? Maybe because it's always been that way—with you desiring sexual intimacy more than your husband. You're in the higher desire sisterhood that's existed through centuries and cultures—part of a long line of sensual women.

Now What?

We've covered a lot of ground, including reasons why your husband might have a lesser drive, how your desire appears higher, and specifics on how to manage various situations.

What I hope you can see, however, is that it's rarely one reason why you and your spouse are mismatched in sexual interest. Like with many other areas of marriage, you may have several aspects to address, work through, heal from, and negotiate with your husband to find unity.

So how do you take all that information and move forward? We'll now address more broadly how you can actively pursue better sexual intimacy.

34. Communicating About Sex

Type "we need to talk memes" into Google Images, and you'll see a slew of pictures showing men with various "oh no!" expressions. Their dread is palpable. But if you changed that to "we need to talk about sex," many men's expressions would go from anxious to eager.

Not so with lower desire husbands. They remain as anxious as before or become even more stressed. After all, they know it's not going well, and they either don't know what to do about it or don't want to face the inevitable pain that comes with working through difficulty.

Starting the Conversation

How can you broach the topic of sex, find common cause, and improve the sexual intimacy in your marriage?

First, recognize that it won't be a single conversation. Years of experience went into developing your views and triggers on these issues, so all the problems won't get resolved on day one. Or day two. Or likely day three.

Consider this conversation as an ongoing one, with stops and starts, breakthroughs and setbacks, revelations and reminders, disagreement and unity. As long as you're making progress on the whole, the conversation is going well.

Here are some tips for setting up the conversation:

- *Wait until you're calm.* Right after he's rejected you sexually, made an unfair demand, or said something hurtful, you're emotionally charged and defensive. Hold off until your heart rate relaxes, your nerves settle, and your mind can focus.

- *Choose a safe location.* The bedroom is usually the wrong place to talk, since his or your emotional baggage might be stored there. Also, while most women connect best when talking face-to-face, men tend to bond shoulder-to-shoulder and open up more during activities that don't require eye contact. It might be more comfortable for your husband to share while walking with you or sitting side by side. Look for neutral ground or a location connected with good feelings for him—whether that's your living room couch, a local park trail, or a fishing boat.

- *Consider time of day.* Attempting to discuss problems when one of you is stressed or weary or angry won't lead to effective listening and problem solving. Set aside time and do your best to figure out which part of the day or week is most likely to result in a fruitful discussion.

- *Give him a heads-up.* Some husbands want or need time to mentally and emotionally prepare, perhaps if only to clear their calendar and minds. If that's your husband, tell him you want to talk about sex—even the specific topic—and ask if the time and place you're suggesting work for him. If not, have him suggest an alternative.

Whenever I say that lower desire spouses can pass on talking about sex at a particular time, higher desire spouses push back, saying their mate won't follow through, so their "not now" turns into never talking about sex. I hear you. Your spouse should have free rein to reschedule a couple of times, but not indefinitely. At some point, you may need to set some boundaries to induce your husband's cooperation.

Once you've both agreed to talk about the issue, prepare your own mind and heart. Take deep breaths to calm yourself. And pray ahead of time.

Now, don't do what I did for years, praying something like, "Lord, please change my husband, because he's the one messing up our marriage." Rather, ask God to direct your thoughts and words, such as, "Lord, please give me an attitude of patience, kindness, and respect, and help me to have words of wisdom as I speak to my husband." Then follow through by accepting his guidance.

Creating a Safe Atmosphere

So you've arrived for this conversation that may last three minutes, thirty minutes, or three hours—depending on the time you have, what exactly you want to discuss, and how it goes. What next?

Most higher desire spouses launch a conversation about sex for two reasons:

1. to resolve the mismatch in sexual interest
2. to express their own hurt and anger

That first goal is laudable. It's the whole point of this book, and I'm rooting for you!

But that second goal? You may not recognize that's what you're doing. You might say you want to "clear the air," "tell you how I really feel," or "be completely honest with you"—when you actually want to feel understood, gain sympathy, and convince your spouse to change.

Do a heart check. Be honest and ask whether that's part of your motivation. If you spend a lot of time on that second selfish goal, you're unlikely to achieve the first excellent goal. Your

223

husband will understandably become defensive and push back or shut down.

If you need to vent, do it! But vent to God, to a trusted friend who supports your marriage, and/or to a counselor, not in the conversation with your husband, whom you need to be vulnerable, open, and cooperative.

With your heart in the right place, here are some tips for creating an atmosphere in which you can both talk freely, negotiate, and resolve problems:

- *Introduce the topic.* State in positive terms what you're seeing as a problem and the process you want to use for fixing it. That could be as simple as "I want us to have sex more frequently, so can we talk about how to reconfigure our schedules to make that happen?" or as complex as "I feel like our sexual intimacy has fallen off lately, and when that happens, it makes me wonder if you're using pornography again, so can we talk about what's happening and how to address it?" Your introduction could also be "I read this book for higher desire wives. One chapter covered something I believe is an issue for us, but I want to know what you think."

- *Ask questions.* Again, as much as you want to express yourself, use this opportunity instead to learn where your husband is coming from. Stephen Covey, author of *7 Habits of Highly Effective People*, said it well with habit 5: "Seek first to understand, then to be understood."[1] Even if you think you've heard it a million times, you probably don't fully understand his background, fears, hurts, dreams, and desires. That involves asking questions.

- *Listen, listen, listen.* Of everything we have to do, this is probably the hardest. We tend to listen to others with the objective of figuring out how we'll reply, and given the subject matter, you may feel triggered at times by what your husband says. But take a deep breath and remember Proverbs 18:13: "To answer before listening—that is folly and shame." Give your husband time and space to explain his perspective and actions, and get comfortable with silence, because it may take him a while to gather his thoughts and his gumption to say what he wants to say.

- *Touch him.* Studies have shown that physical affection lowers stress by decreasing blood pressure, heart rate, and the stress hormone cortisol and also by releasing oxytocin. So, if he's amenable, hold his hand, stroke his chest, arm, or thigh, or snuggle as you talk.

- *Avoid assumptions and conclusions.* Some of the biggest disagreements in my marriage happened when one of us reacted negatively to what we *thought* the other was saying when they weren't saying that at all. If it feels to you like your husband is saying X when he says Y, don't assume. Rather . . .

- *Ask for clarification.* Check your understanding of what he's saying. Repeat back what you heard. Ask follow-up questions. Even say, "I'm not sure what you mean. Can you tell me more?" Make sure you're receiving the message he's sending.

- *Focus on intimacy.* Too often, lower desire spouses hear that their mate wants more sex without understanding that their mate's real longing is to feel desired, connected, loved. Express what having sex really means to you deep down. Sure, it feels good, but if it were only about a physical release of tension, let's face it: you could do that yourself. Instead, you desire to be one with your spouse, so communicate that.

- *Deal with the issue at hand.* When you're in the midst of conflict, it's all too easy to default to "and another thing . . ." and drag in unrelated infractions, or make statements with "always" and "never," such as "You never care about what I want!" Most husbands will react by building emotional walls to protect their hearts. Instead, choose one area where you want to start improving your sexual intimacy and focus on that.

- *Look for common ground.* When you're on the same page about something, take a moment to acknowledge that. Even celebrate it. Too many times, we're so concerned about closing the gaps, we don't recognize the unity we have. Indeed, studies show that many spouses both want more sex in their marriage; they just disagree about how to get there.

- *Take a "we" attitude.* It's always easier to talk about our personal failings with someone we know has our back. Make it clear that you're in your husband's corner, wanting to be a united, one-flesh couple as you work through issues. That doesn't mean you can't set boundaries—that may be the right choice—but frame the conversation as a team effort to fight back against whatever has compromised your marital intimacy.

As neuroscientists have noted, our need for safety is deeply wired into our minds and bodies. It's when we feel emotionally safe that we can be vulnerable, trust one another, and pursue deep intimacy.[2] Use these tips to promote emotional safety and work toward the sexual intimacy you want for your marriage.

Asking for Changes

The first, second, or fifth conversation may not be the one where you ask for changes. You may be on a fact-finding mission for a while—gathering information about what's going on, how your husband views the problem, where you're in unity, and where you're in conflict. Or it may be clear from day one that a particular thing needs to go differently.

Whichever way it goes, how can you ask for changes in a way that encourages follow-through? Here are some suggestions:

- *Go first.* Own whatever you've done poorly in this situation, even if it's just your obvious frustration, and offer to make some changes on your end. Even if your husband is 95% responsible for the difficulties in your marital intimacy, you can tackle that last 5%. Ask your husband what one step you could take that would mean so much to him. As long as it's not against God's will or your conscience, commit to doing it.

- *Cast a vision.* Instead of concentrating on what's gone wrong, talk about what you want your sex life to be. What would it look like for you and your husband to thrive in this area of your marriage? Look ahead to a positive future rather than dwelling on problems in the past.

- *Ask for baby steps.* Most of us have reasons why we haven't already made the changes we should. To get past that natural reluctance and onto the right path, simply start with the next step. What's one thing your husband could do to improve the situation? Make a doctor's appointment? Add one sexual encounter to your monthly schedule? Initiate sometime in the next couple of weeks? Prioritize moving in the right direction, and over time you can make a lot of progress.

- *Set a follow-up.* Let him know you want to reconvene from time to time to see how it's going, how you can better support one another, what the next step might be, etc. Then ask when you can meet again. This shouldn't come across as an accountability session so much as checking in and encouraging one another toward greater intimacy.

- *Help him stay focused.* If your husband tends not to follow through, ask how he'd like to make sure it happens. Would he like you to remind him? If so, how? Or should he schedule reminders on his calendar or put Post-its on his mirror? Avoid nagging him, but rather acknowledge that it's hard for him to remember and offer to help so that this endeavor can succeed.

Change takes time. But in a covenant marriage, we have the time to make great strides toward fostering intimacy if we take the journey step-by-step. Use these suggestions to help you get going and to maintain progress.

Making the Changes Last

You won't fix your issues once and be done with it. Everyone I know who's had fantastic sexual intimacy in their marriage has also had speed bumps from time to time.

Ideally, these conversations become a habit in your marriage, as you learn to talk about sexual intimacy more openly and effectively. You check in with each other to ask how it's going, talk about what you're seeing and feeling, and come up with next steps to take. Anticipating periodic problems and having a growth mindset can help you weather the mists and storms of your marriage.

One great resource for having quality conversations about sex, now and for the rest of your marriage, is my book *Pillow Talk: 40 Conversations About Sex for Married Couples.* Many couples have reported that it took the pressure off to go through this comprehensive guide. But whether you go for my resource or another, the point is to learn how to talk about sexual intimacy. Such conversations can feel awkward at first, but they yield high dividends when you become comfortable with them in your marriage.

When He Won't Talk or Act

All these suggestions presume your husband will engage in these conversations. However, every time I suggest communicating with a spouse about sex, someone tells me they've tried and their mate just won't do it. Any attempt to start a conversation is met with silence, absence, or anger.

If that's where you are, I recommend telling your husband that you're not giving up—that healthy and holy sexual intimacy in your marriage matters. But that doesn't mean you should keep talking about it. Continuing to push a conversation with an unwilling person can result in them shutting down even more.

You may want to give your husband a break. Step away for a while, pray and work on your own issues, and wait until things are calmer before broaching the subject again. That time away could be what's needed for you both to get perspective.

You may also want to seek therapy for your own hurt and for ideas on how to proceed. A counselor who knows about your particular situation can support you and offer tailored advice. If your husband is willing to attend therapy with you, that's great. Sometimes a spouse is motivated to go when they know or suspect they're going to be talked about, and sliding into the appointment gives them an opportunity to share their side. But pursue the counseling you and your marriage need.

You may wish to set some boundaries as well. What are boundaries? They are lines that you draw in the sand along with specific, calm consequences you'll follow through on if the other person steps over the line. They're not ultimatums or punishments but rather choices you make to keep yourself (and your husband) physically and emotionally safe. One quick example: "If you call me sex-crazed again, I'm leaving the room because I won't let myself be belittled that way." I highly recommend Henry Cloud and John Townsend's book *Boundaries in Marriage* for more on how to set boundaries well.

In the end, however, engaging sexually is and should be an individual choice. You can't force it, and pressuring your husband into sex won't build intimacy in the long run. You can't even force your husband to talk about it with you. If you push too hard, you may get a back-and-forth, but in the form of a fight, not a conversation.

Contrast these two passages:

> Better to live on a corner of the roof
>   than share a house with a quarrelsome wife. (Prov. 21:9)

> Houses and wealth are inherited from parents,
>   but a prudent wife is from the LORD. (Prov. 19:14)

A husband wants distance from a quarrelsome wife, while a prudent wife is better than houses or wealth, yielding far more for a husband in his lifetime.

A frustrated higher desire wife—a wife who longs for the sexual intimacy God desires her marriage to have—can be tempted to be quarrelsome. But remember your husband's free will. Use your influence. You have a lot of that, prudent wife! Keep working toward something better, but be wise and measured in how you go about it.

Meanwhile, invest in your own health, friendships, and relationship with God. Even if your sex life isn't quite where you'd like it to be, you can find great joy and comfort in these things, as well as a reminder of your value.

35. Engaging Your Husband

Some movie scenes stick with you, even if they have little impact on others. In *She's the One*, Jennifer Aniston plays a wife whose husband has rejected her sexually, and following advice from others, she freshens up, dons a slinky nightgown, and seductively slides into bed.

For most men, a clear offer from Jennifer Aniston would be met with YES! But her husband, played by Michael McGlone, doesn't even look up from his laptop. She might as well be a fluff pillow on the bed, hardly worth noticing and easily tossed aside.

That movie came out in 1996, yet I remember the scene well. Because I knew the feeling and the bad advice that led there. Higher desire wives are often advised to ramp up their sexual advances, make their offer clear and their lingerie sheer, and expect an eager husband—only to feel even worse when their extra efforts are rebuffed.

What works for lower desire wives often doesn't work for higher desire wives, not because those wives aren't sexually appealing but because their husbands respond to different stimuli. How can you engage your lower desire guy?

Responsive Desire

For decades, scientists and practitioners viewed the sexual cycle as following a standard progression:

- desire—wanting sex
- arousal—physiological stimulation
- orgasm—*woot woot!*
- resolution—return to equilibrium

Until 2011, when researcher Rosemary Basson said, "Whoa, wait a minute!" (I paraphrase) and suggested that many women don't start with desire.[1] Rather, their desire kicks in sometime after becoming aroused. To which many wives proclaimed, "Exactly!" and a new paradigm was born.

Basson proposed that some sexual partners had a spontaneous desire and others were responsive. Other terms for those include initiating and receptive desire—the main issue being, which happens first, desire or arousal? And those categories are not strictly divided by gender; some wives feel desire before sexual initiation and some husbands don't get into it until sexual initiation has begun.

For many men, this is a big shift in thinking. It never occurred to them before that they might be a more responsive lover. They assumed falling in love with a woman and wanting to connect with her equaled assertive sexual desire. But not necessarily. It's A-OK for a husband to respond to sexual arousal rather than pursue it. That doesn't diminish his love or interest in being with his wife.

Start with the notion that it's okay for him to be the receptive partner. That's not a demerit on his love card but rather the way he's built.

Ready for Romance

Reams and reams of paper have been spent telling husbands to romance their wives. But plenty of husbands long for romance too. Mind you, it may not look like the romance women want, but a bit of wooing can go a long way for many lower desire husbands.

How would your husband define romance? Ask him what revs his romance engine, makes him feel loved, and gets him excited about being with you.

Tailor romance to your particular mate. My own husband finds a shared game of table tennis more romantic than a candle-light dinner. But whether it's mutual recreation, physical affection, or something else, home in on what reaches out to your guy's heart.

Clear the Obstacles

What's in the way of your husband's sex drive? Hopefully, you've been able to pinpoint some options as you've read this book. Once you know what those obstacles are, can you help him clear them?

For instance, if stress is the major roadblock to sexual desire, could you step up and help him to get perspective or to let go of some of his emotional burden? If he's not eating well, could you help him identify better choices and shop accordingly? Smoothing that path for your husband could make him more willing to step out and engage sexually.

I'm not saying you should twist yourself into a hard knot to make his life easy! You have your own stress, and it isn't your job to fix your spouse. As his *ezer* (Hebrew for "powerful help"—see Gen. 2:18), partner *with* your husband to remove roadblocks that keep him from being fully present and sexually interested.

Be His Wife

Now and then, I hear from a higher desire wife who's identified the problems, informed her husband, introduced changes, and held him accountable. After all her heroic efforts, she wonders why he still isn't eager to have sex.

If I could sit down with the husband, I might hear that he finds his wife attractive and wants to have sex with her—if only she'd stop micromanaging him. With his every step numbered and measured, his wife feels more like a mother. And no sane man wants to have sex with his mother.

Other roles you play in marriage can turn off a willing, even receptive husband, such as administrative assistant, household manager, and 24/7 mom to your kids. Of course you wear many hats in your life! But in your direct relationship with your husband, remember that you're his wife.

Neither of you should be the other's boss. (If he thinks he's your boss, you have marital problems beyond sexuality; seek help.) Rather, you should be each other's life partner, lover, and friend.

Nurture the Relationship

Speaking of being a friend, one of the best investments any higher desire spouse can make for a lower desire spouse is nurturing their relationship outside the bedroom. Lower desire spouses want—even need—to feel valued as a person before they can appreciate their value as a lover.

Do you and your husband spend time as a couple? Do you have shared interests or activities? Do you have nonsexual touch throughout the day? Do you talk well and laugh together? Do you communicate about who you really are, not just about schedules and people you know?

If you've lost that lovin' feelin', consider how to get back to the couple that fell in love. Mind you, it won't feel the same, because falling in love the first time stimulates the release of butterfly-in-your-tummy body chemicals, while falling further in love stimulates the release of warmth-in-your-chest body chemicals. Both are wonderful feelings but different.

How can you prioritize your relationship? Here are some ideas:

- regular date nights (out or in)
- daily check-ins to see how you're each doing
- walking the neighborhood hand in hand
- trying a new activity together
- twenty-second embraces (that length releases oxytocin)
- praying together
- ten- to fifteen-minute conversations on get-to-know-you topics

If you want help getting started, you can find devotional books and conversation starters at Christian bookstores, from online ministries, and perhaps in your church library. Those can launch some great discussions and greater connection.

Be Available

Given my ministry addressing sex in marriage, I understand the sex drive spectrum better than most, yet I experienced my own share of disappointment when I initiated sex and got a "no thanks" from my stressed and sapped husband. Having put myself out there, I felt slapped down and scooted away.

None of that was his intention, but it was how it felt to me. Perhaps you can relate.

Then I came up with an approach that worked so much better for us. Rather than suggesting sex, I let my husband know I was available. For instance: "I'd be up for sex tonight. I'm headed to bed soon, and if you're interested, join me."

Without directly initiating, I didn't feel any expectation. And because I wasn't saying, "Do you want to?" I didn't hear "no."

Meanwhile, he didn't feel any pressure. It was an offer he could take or leave, which made it more appealing to him.

He still passed sometimes, but flipping the switch from initiation to availability increased our sexual frequency and decreased our tension. All of which strengthened our sexual intimacy.

Ask for Rain Checks

When it comes to sex, the word "no" can feel like a wallop in the chest. As I noted in chapter 32, what feels so much better is "not now."

After all, even stuff we absolutely adore, we don't want any minute of the day. I'm a huge fan of roller coasters, waterslides, and line dancing, but I'm not game for them after a big meal. And good gravy, do not disturb my sleep to get me to do any of those!

Encourage your husband to use the phrase "not now" rather than "no." And if he says either of those, ask when might be better. You might be surprised to discover that your husband has ideas on a better time for him to get in the mood. Or maybe his time window is a bit vaguer, but he's at least more open to the idea, knowing that he gets to help choose the when.

A rain check might be as simple as "after I finish this task," a specific date and time, or sometime in the next day or so. Be flexible about when the rain check can be cashed, but it should be within a few days.

What if your husband doesn't honor the rain check? Remind him what he suggested, but don't pressure or force it. You can have a bigger discussion later about follow-through, but getting mad in the moment isn't likely to lead to more sex. If your husband doesn't keep his promises in this and other things, once again, you may have other problems in your marriage that need addressing.

Celebrate Successes

Has your husband made any positive changes in the sex department? Acknowledge them with a simple thanks or by sharing how good his efforts make you feel. We're motivated to keep making progress if and when we believe our previous efforts have yielded good results.

Engaging your husband isn't as easy as wearing a teddy, and that's all right. You'll both grow as you learn to decode one another's makeup and create marital intimacy that's satisfying for both of you and can weather the storms of life.

36. Initiating Intimacy

We've talked about engaging your husband generally, but how can you effectively start a single sexual encounter? How can you initiate in a way that appeals to your husband, arouses his interest, and actually gets him to show up in the bedroom?

As you've seen from all the reasons why a husband might be less interested than his wife, there's no magic formula. No guarantee. If there was, I'd share it with you. I'd use it myself! But I've learned a thing or two about increasing the odds that he'll engage.

Let's talk first about what doesn't work and then what might work when it comes to initiating sex with a lower desire husband.

Sexy Doesn't Do It

Some of the standard advice given to wives to initiate with their husbands includes:

- Just walk into the room wearing sexy lingerie or nothing.
- Pull him into a passionate kiss or cup his crotch.
- Be straightforward about wanting sex, like saying, "I want you, right now."
- On your next date, skip wearing panties and then tell him you're undies-free.
- Whisper in his ear what you want to do with or to him.

Perhaps you tried one or more of these and discovered they don't work. That's because they presume an equally matched or higher desire husband. But imagine if men tried comparable approaches with lower desire wives. What would the success rate be? It wouldn't be high.

That's why men aren't generally given this advice. Rather, higher desire husbands are encouraged to create opportunities, extend invitations, and help their lower desire spouse become aroused. Not bad advice for HDWs either, although the form that takes is different because, well, your husband's a man and you're a woman.

Pushing Can Push Him Away

When an HDW pushes for sex with her husband—through frequent initiation, constantly bringing up the subject, pleading or yelling about not getting sex, etc.—her efforts can backfire. It's understandable that you're in a place of internal turmoil and ache for something to change. But your husband may end up feeling under pressure and turn to ice ice baby.

Ideally, he'd see what you're really saying and feeling, but the truth is that your requests, pleas, and demands may overwhelm him. You may need to dial down your intensity, give him more space to breathe, and learn how to approach him more calmly.

And yes, this means *you* have to be the one to make more adjustments, because it's a topic you care about more *and* I have your ear instead of his.

Taking Over Can Undermine

Deborah Tannen, linguist and author of *You Just Don't Understand Me*, has studied gender communication extensively. She points out that men's conversational rituals are often about information and status, while women's conversations are about relationship.

Walking away from the same conversation, women and men may have different interpretations. And often, it's because the women are focusing on the question of connection. *Is this way of speaking bringing us closer or pulling us further apart?* Meanwhile, men are coming to the same conversation looking at a different axis, a different question. *Is this conversation putting one of us in a one-up or one-down position?*[1]

Tannen's work is based primarily on studying children, meaning these communication patterns manifest from a very early age. But they continue into adulthood.

What that means is that men can be extra-sensitive to status in the relationship. This sensitivity can be heightened when a wife becomes more assertive sexually. Although her intention is bringing the couple closer, he may read it as undermining his position in the marriage. It can feel like her taking over, thus lowering his value, perhaps in her eyes but definitely in his own.

The answer is not to say nothing, do nothing, be a wallflower, and wait for your husband to make a move. However, be aware of how your pursuit of intimacy can be misread and make sure that, while being proactive, you're not coming across as aggressive or undermining his manhood.

Take the Pressure Off

One specific way to lower the pressure and minimize status issues is to come up with a low-tension signal for sexual initiation. I don't claim credit for these ideas, as they've been shared widely by authors, therapists, pastors, and others who work with couples. But among the suggested signals are:

- Use pillows that read "Yes" on one side and "No" on the other, and flip your pillows according to your willingness to have sex that day or night.
- Light a bedside candle to indicate your desire.

- Use a code word, euphemism, or symbol to communicate sexual interest.
- Go to bed naked as a show of immediate desire.

None of these requires bringing up the topic, initiating in a way that may feel like cornering to a lower desire spouse, or making a direct bid that could be rejected. They do require you each agreeing to the signaling system, but if you read the previous chapter on communicating about sex, hopefully that's in your wheelhouse.

Schedule Sex

Every time I suggest scheduling sex, someone balks at the idea. *Whatever happened to romance? Passion? Spontaneity?* And then I point out that they used to schedule dates, right?

Before marriage, most of us lined up a specific day and time to see our romantic partner, then boyfriend, and finally fiancé. He might have asked you out for "Friday night at 7:00 p.m." or just texted earlier in the day to say, "Wanna hang out tonight?" Both of those were scheduling time to be with one another. Just like you can do with sex.

Scheduling sex simply means finding a time that works for both of you and doing your best to show up at that time for physical intimacy. You're not scheduling exactly what happens once you get there. You can have plenty of spontaneity with positions, activities, etc. But scheduling takes away the higher desire spouse's anxiety of wondering when they'll have sex again, while the lower desire spouse gets time to prepare mentally, emotionally, and physically.

Some couples have a standing date each week, like every Wednesday evening or Saturday morning. Other couples check in with each other a day or two ahead of when they want to have sex. Yet others reserve a window of days for sex to happen. My husband and I do a fair amount of "how's your day looking?" to see if sex might work on a particular day.

Talk to your husband about scheduling at least a couple of sexual encounters per month. And remember that scheduled events sometimes don't happen, but having them on the calendar makes them more likely to.

Score Brownie Points

I've compared wanting sex to my love of brownies. This was before I discovered a food sensitivity that has required me to knock out all sugar (dear God, why?!).

> I eat when I'm hungry (internal) and when someone places a brownie in front of me (external). . . .
>
> Your words and actions can be external factors (like brownies) that make him more likely to want to have sex (eat). You want to be the kind of wife that would draw a husband closer. In essence, you want to Be the Brownie.[2]

I went on to discuss that "Be the Brownie" did not mean "just look sexy, throw yourself at your husband, etc."[3] Not only does that not get you to full sexual intimacy, but it usually doesn't work in HDW/LDH marriages. Rather, it's about being the sort of person that piques his interest and encourages contact.

I purposefully called this chapter "initiating intimacy" instead of "initiating sex" because that approach has a better likelihood of success. Pursuing companionship, showing interest in what matters to him, reassuring your hubby of your admiration and love, and investing in other forms of intimacy—emotional, spiritual, intellectual, recreational—can lay the groundwork for physical intimacy.

When you show that you want *all* of him, your lower desire husband is more likely to bring his sexual self to you as well.

242

Ask Him to Get Things Started

Sadly, many lower desire husbands feel they aren't as manly as they should be. Most of this comes from societal pressure, but you can add to or ease it with how you address your own husband.

One option is simply to ask him to step up and initiate when he's interested or willing. Tony and Alisa DiLorenzo, hosts of the ONE *Extraordinary Marriage* podcast, have long suggested taking turns initiating, with the husband and wife each making a bid once a week. Of course, this requires follow-through, which may or may not be your husband's strong suit.

But giving your husband a window of a few days to initiate could help him feel like more of a participant in sexual intimacy. It could give him the opportunity to explore when he's most up for things and how he likes sexual intimacy to unfold. It can be hard to wait on him during that time, but if he can step up and initiate in the time you both agreed to, it will be good for your marriage.

And remember, one failure doesn't mean the whole idea is doomed. If he misses an encounter, gently remind him, but then lay off and see if he steps up the next time.

Be Blunt

After all my suggestions about not being blunt, how can I now suggest that you be blunt? Because sometimes it's a good idea. Again, this depends on what's hindering your sex life and how your particular husband sees the issue. But sometimes just saying, "Hey, I want to have sex. Wanna give it a shot?" yields a fantastic sexual experience.

Some lower desire husbands dislike hints, discussion, and guessing about sex and would rather you just say what you want. Then he can say yes or no, but he'll give more yeses when you're direct.

Ask your husband which approach he prefers—indirect, direct, or something in between. His preference might depend on time and mood. But it's worth asking what kind of initiation he would like from you.

Experiment with the Formula

There's no easy fix, but experiment with various approaches to see how they might work in your marriage. One suggestion above might be great for couple A and another for couple B. Don't worry about the ones that aren't a fit. Just keep your eyes on the goal of figuring out which ones are helpful to your marriage.

37. Dealing with Rejection

I once asked my higher desire wife community what emotions they felt when their husband turned down sex. Here are just a few of the feelings they shared:

anxious
betrayed
disappointed
embarrassed
frustrated
lonely
oversensitive
pushy
selfish
undesirable
unloved
unwanted[1]

When higher desire spouses who've been regularly refused send me messages, their emotional pain pops off the page. While their lower desire spouses might believe it's about the physical act of sex, it's not. They don't feel their offer for a fun activity has been rejected, but rather a core part of themselves.

Higher desire wives can feel this pain even more intensely because they were set up to believe that husbands desire all but the worst wives. By now, I pray you know this is not true, but it can take time for your feelings to catch up with your knowledge. You can help yourself get there by coming up with a plan of how to cope with your emotions.

So how can you deal with the pangs of rejection?

Feel Free to Grieve

Scripture offers us some powerful and moving verses about grief. Consider just a few:

My heart has turned to wax;
  it has melted within me. (Ps. 22:14)

Joy is gone from our hearts;
  our dancing has turned to mourning. (Lam. 5:15)

My soul is overwhelmed with sorrow to the point of death. (Matt. 26:38)

Verses like these aren't the ones we memorize. We'd rather stick with the likes of "For God so loved the world that he gave his one and only Son, that whoever believes in him shall not perish but have eternal life" (John 3:16), and "'For I know the plans I have for you,' declares the LORD, 'plans to prosper you and not to harm you, plans to give you a hope and a future'" (Jer. 29:11). Yes, we'll take that love, eternal life, hope, and future.

And yet, grief is common in God's Word. As people experienced loss and disappointment, they voiced their hurt—to God and to others. Grief is biblical.

Christians must reclaim the power of lament—including over lost moments of marital intimacy, a spouse's sexual rejection, and heartache from not feeling fully desired by the one you desire. Cry out to God. Share with fellow believers who'll hold your pain with honor and root for your marriage. Express your hurt, your fears, your sense of hopelessness.

It's easy to brush our feelings aside, to think we don't have time to cry. For some of us, grief can feel self-indulgent. But it's not. Our feelings are real, and they matter.

If you need a safe place to grieve, check out my higher desire wife community (HDWives.HotHolyHumorous.com). We will mourn with you, empathize with you, and pray for you.

Remember Compassion

Years ago, when my husband and I were going through the worst time in our marriage, we played the dynamic of pursuer-distancer over and over again. Our issues then weren't about sex, but I would bring up problems in our relationship, eager to discuss our concerns and wanting to push through conflict to resolution. (Pursuer.) My husband, meanwhile, became emotionally flooded at the first flare of conflict and shut down. (Distancer.)

Why doesn't he care? I'd ask myself. *Does he even love me?*

With many years of hindsight, I can answer those questions with yes, he cared, and yes, he loved me. But he was hurting too, and bringing up issues he didn't know how to fix made him feel even worse. Once I began to have compassion for his emotional pain, I felt less alone.

Later, when my sex drive topped his (by a mountain mile), it took me a while to remember that when we weren't connecting well—whether relationally or sexually—he was hurting too. Although he was the one saying no, we were both missing out.

Your husband likely isn't saying no because he doesn't love you. Rather, he has sexual baggage, physical or emotional challenges, or another obstacle in the way of engaging sexually more often and more fully. Remember to have compassion for him.

Compassion doesn't excuse behavior, but it reminds us we're not alone. After all, marriage bonds us together, so that when one of us hurts, it impacts both of us. We sink or rise together.

Release Tension

Some HDWs have so much pent-up energy, they feel like an overly tight guitar string: one hard pluck and—*splang!*—they'll break. Since I (once again, so sadly) can't guarantee you'll get sex in the near future, you may need to find a way to expend some of that energy. It won't sate your desire for intimacy with your husband, but it can keep you from coming apart.

Here are some positive outlets for the stress that builds inside when you don't have sexual release:

- *Get moving.* What if the next time you got all hot and bothered, you took a run? Went to a dance class? Pummeled a punching bag? Physical activity can release sexual tension, and it's also good for your physical and mental health. If I'm left in the lurch a couple times too many, you might find me gyrating around my living room like a music video backup dancer—or my middle-aged, never-enter-a-contest version of it.
- *Try a creative hobby.* Anything from knitting to painting to writing a book. (Trust me, writing an entire book takes energy.)
- *Plan an adventure.* Take a day trip to someplace new or knock out a bucket list item.
- *Get with friends who make you laugh.* Proverbs 17:22 says, "A cheerful heart is good medicine, but a broken spirit saps a person's strength" (NLT). Don't ignore your spirit, but counteract that sense of brokenness with cheerfulness wherever and however you can find it.

- *Engage in self-care.* That could mean a spa day, ordering dessert, or spending an afternoon reading. Find an activity that eases your mind and soul and make it a priority.
- *Take on a new project.* I had a friend who released the tension of infertility by gardening; when she and her husband couldn't produce children, they still produced beauty in their landscape beds. You might refurbish a room, rebuild a car, or organize a charity drive. But find a project that gives you pleasure in both process and product.

By prioritizing your well-being and activities that release energy and bring joy, you can find better emotional balance and an ability to cope with the disappointments of life.

What About Masturbation?

Speaking of relieving tension, one of the most common questions higher desire wives ask is whether it's okay to masturbate when they've gone a long time without sex. My answer is . . . it depends.

Consider your own theological beliefs about masturbation. Do you believe it's okay with God? Many Catholic friends would say it's sin. Other friends who've struggled with pornography, erotica, or solo masturbation would say it's unwise. And still others would say it's fine. Based on my study, I don't believe all masturbation is sinful or perfectly fine, but there's wise and unwise use of it.

Masturbation can be self-indulgent and take energy from the marriage bed. Engaging in regular masturbation, especially if it involves porn or fantasies of others, can become a crutch or add to frustration with a partner. A woman who masturbates might experience an increased sense of sexual urgency, find it easier to get herself to climax than pitch a sexual encounter to her husband that may or may not happen, and even become desensitized to her husband's touch. It can alter her view of sexual arousal and orgasm to be a more selfish activity than an opportunity to bond with her husband.

But masturbation could help sexual intimacy with a spouse. Some wives have benefited from touching themselves to learn what feels good so they can better teach their husband what to do when he touches her. Other spouses in long-distance relationships have reported getting on the phone or a video call and using simultaneous solo masturbation to have a mutual encounter that feels connecting for both. And yet others have been able to give more grace to a partner unable or unwilling to engage when they "take the edge off."

Consider your reasons for masturbation, how frequently you might use it, how you're doing it, and how you're working on your sex life with your husband. Masturbation should not be a substitute for addressing issues in your marriage bed. But it might be an okay practice to release some tension and allow you to fight another day.

Again, if you believe masturbation is sinful, find other ways to release that tension. "For you are not following your convictions. If you do anything you believe is not right, you are sinning" (Rom. 14:23 NLT).

Pursue Happiness

When your sex life or marriage isn't all it could be, you can feel consumed by those struggles. But your identity is not wrapped up entirely in your sexuality. You can soothe the wounds of rejection by finding other ways to satisfy your longing for sensual pleasure and connection with others.

One of the most effective ways to cope with perceived rejection is to pursue happiness independent of your husband. What brightens your day? What eases your stress? What makes you smile or laugh? What helps you feel more alive?

Your joyous moments could involve anything from a girls' night out to a solo fly-fishing trip. I'm partial to reading novels and singing at the top of my lungs. But as my Gen Z sons say, you do you.

The truth is, becoming a happier wife is a gift not just to yourself but also to your husband and to your marriage. Happy people are attractive people. Joy draws others in like the smell of chocolate chip cookies baking in the oven. It's not selfish to seek joy in your life. Quite the contrary. It can be a key to helping you deal with rejection and inviting your husband closer.

Embrace Your Beauty

I've never met an HDW who didn't strike me as gorgeous. No, my standards aren't limbo-bar low. Rather, I see these women and immediately understand why their husbands chose them.

Even more so, I see why God loves them. Every wife is made in the image of God with lovely traits that reflect his glory. Every wife has unique features that reveal aspects of him worth knowing. Every wife has her own story worth hearing. Every wife was once a hopeful bride. As Isaiah 62:5 says, "As a bridegroom rejoices over his bride, so will your God rejoice over you."

The Song of Songs husband calls his wife "most beautiful of women" (1:8), yet when your husband rejects your sexual advances, you may feel anything but beautiful. Don't believe the lie. Embrace your beauty—as seen and known by your Creator, your Savior, your heavenly husband.

Remind yourself that you're "worth more than many sparrows" (Luke 12:7). God doesn't make dogs-playing-poker art. He makes masterpieces. And you, dear woman, are one.

38. Embracing Your Desire

If I had ten bucks for every time a higher desire spouse told me that they wished their sex drive would go away, I'd be vacationing in Greece right now. It's common for sexually frustrated husbands and wives to imagine that life would be easier if they didn't care so much about being physically intimate with their mate. They envision a marriage without the irritation, resentment, and loneliness that come with not feeling intensely desired.

Emotionally, I relate. When you're in pain, you just want the pain to stop.

Logically, I disagree. Pain often exists to inform you that something needs to be fixed. Even if you don't currently know how to fix it. Even if it might not be fixed.

Spiritually, I object. God often speaks to us most clearly when we feel broken and in (desperate) need of rescue. He also refines our character in the fire of adversity. "See, I have refined you, though not as silver; I have tested you in the furnace of affliction" (Isa. 48:10). Our pain could be his opening to make us more like him.

> We also glory in our sufferings, because we know that suffering produces perseverance; perseverance, character; and character, hope. And hope does not put us to shame, because God's love has been poured out into our hearts through the Holy Spirit, who has been given to us. (Rom. 5:3–5)

But yeah, I feel ya. This is not an easy road to walk. Sometimes it's all you can do to put one foot in front of the other and hang in there for another week, day, or minute.

I Thank God for You

In his letter to the Christians in Colossae, the apostle Paul wrote, "We always thank God, the Father of our Lord Jesus Christ, when we pray for you, because we have heard of your faith in Christ Jesus and of the love you have for all God's people" (Col. 1:3–4).

His sentiment is how I feel about higher desire wives. I assume that you also have faith in Christ Jesus and love for God's people, that those are more important than sex, but also that part of the love Jehovah God affirms is sexual love in marriage. Bonding with your beloved mate through this intimate knowing of one another's bodies conforms with God's will. And you can be thankful that at least one of you understands how important that type of intimacy is.

If not for you, what would happen to sex in your marriage? Would it stop? Happen rarely? Fade into the background—a distant memory of what had happened once upon a time? How would that benefit your marriage?

It wouldn't.

As difficult as it is to be sexually frustrated, it would be worse to be sexually absent. Your whole marriage would suffer from having no one advocating for greater physical intimacy.

If you're the one keeping hope for something better alive, that's a good thing. A healthy thing. A grace thing. Thank God.

You're Sexual, Duh

Healthy people are sexual people. They're aware of their sensuality and desire for intimate physical contact. They long to be "one flesh" with a single individual with whom they share life and love.

Whether your husband faces sexual interest obstacles or just happens to be less interested than you, it's good and healthy for you to want to have sex with him. God planted that desire in you. If I've quoted it once, I've quoted it a hundred times:

> For you created my inmost being;
>   you knit me together in my mother's womb.
> I praise you because I am fearfully and wonderfully made;
>   your works are wonderful,
>   I know that full well. (Ps. 139:13–14)

It wasn't a mistake that God made you a sexual being. Accept his craftsmanship. Embrace his artistry. Own your God-given desire.

And use it to make your marriage better—for both of you.

It's Not Fair

Because you have this desire, the burden to pursue regular, mutually satisfying sexual intimacy has fallen on you. Is that fair? Absolutely not.

But if you want to use a scorecard to measure your marriage, you might as well give up now. That way madness lies. All aspects of marriage cannot be distributed in a perfect 50-50 split, and it's likely your husband carries more of the burden in some other area. Hopefully, he doesn't view that as unfair, because a healthy relationship often involves contributing in areas that best suit your abilities and desires.

Again, your husband likely cannot understand how deeply the issue of sex affects you. Most lower desire husbands are not malicious so much as clueless. It's like how my husband leaves shoes out. I used to trip on them, grumble to myself about how inconsiderate he was, and let him know that he'd injured me. He didn't even notice his shoes were out, wasn't putting them there to peeve me, and bristled when I pointed out his colossal mistake. After a while, I realized it mattered far more to me than to him, and—as unfair as it was—I had to take the lead in correcting the situation. I began to pick up his shoes, toss them in the closet, and move on. Once I let go of my need to convince him he was wrong, wrong, wrong, things calmed down. Eventually, I could say to him, "Hey, could you put these shoes away?" without animus or conflict. When I began to make my request more casually, he typically took care of it right away.

Unless you're in an abusive or emotionally destructive marriage, your husband isn't targeting you for sexual rejection. Admittedly, it isn't fair that you're hurting from his lack of interest. Still, you can decide how you'll respond. Will you remain in the "It's unfair!" rant camp? Or own your desire while helping your husband increase his?

Standing in the Gap

Ezekiel was a prophet among the Jewish exiles during Babylonian captivity. While reviewing the fall of Jerusalem in 586 BC, Ezekiel shared one of God's reasons for allowing his people to be overtaken: "I looked for someone among them who would build up the wall and stand before me in the gap on behalf of the land so I would not have to destroy it, but I found no one" (Ezek. 22:30). The gap isn't literal but rather a metaphor for defending God's people against danger.[1]

Imagine an ancient wall with a gap in it, a few stones that crumbled and left a vulnerability. Without someone standing in the gap, defending the weak spot, an enemy could pierce the defenses and attack the residents within.

That wall is your marriage. Any number of issues can create a gap that the enemy would love to wriggle through to destroy your covenant before God. One major issue is sexual intimacy, and the mismatch of desire constitutes a gap. Your longing for something

255

better, for a repair in that wall, could be what's keeping your marital defenses strong. Are you prepared to stand in the gap?

Embrace your desire. Embrace your calling. Embrace God's plan.

I cannot guarantee that the wall will be rebuilt stronger than before. But I can guarantee that God knows your longings. He wants you to embrace your desire and do what you can to strengthen your marriage.

39. FAQs for HDWs

Through blog comments and emails, conversations and interviews, and my communities, I've heard from hundreds of higher desire wives, and certain questions get asked again and again. In this chapter, we'll tackle those frequently asked questions and come up with some answers.

How Can I Connect with Other HDWs?

You've read about how 20–25% of marriages involve a higher desire wife, but if that's true, where are they?! Because everywhere you turn, you feel outnumbered.

In my personal life, outside my ministry, I've discovered other higher desire wives by being the first to fess up. Sometimes when I speak about my higher sex drive, I get pushback or even mocking from other wives, but other times I find curiosity or an ally facing the same challenge. It's risky, but the reward has been worth it to discover compatriots. And to those who don't get it, "forgive them, for they do not know what they do" (Luke 23:34 NKJV).

If you choose to speak, please don't give a barbed complaint about your husband, but rather recognize the sex drive dynamics in your marriage. Share your struggles, ask for encouragement, and support other wives in their struggles.

Also, as I've mentioned, I maintain an online subscription community for higher desire wives who want to get to know others in the same boat. If you want to get connected, head to my website (HotHolyHumorous.com) and find the link to check us out.

How Often Should We Be Having Sex?

Most mentors—therapists, pastors, ministry folk like me—shy away from answering this question directly. They'll say things like, "Every relationship is different, and what matters most is that you're both okay with the frequency."

But I'll just say it: at least once a week. That's what scads of research have told us is best for our marriage and our bodies. Regular sex has many health and relationship benefits, and you don't get those without engaging about once a week.[1]

That frequency won't be sustainable in certain seasons of your life—such as after pregnancy, while apart for an extended period of time (for example, military deployment), or during health difficulties. But once a week is a good goal. And if you and your husband want to have sex more often, go ahead! As Song of Songs 5:1 says, "Drink your fill of love."

Is God Punishing Me?

Some wives wonder if the sexual desire gap in their marriage is God sticking it to them for something they did wrong in their past. That's not what's happening. Even when we experience the consequences of our own sin, God's not leaning over us with his arms crossed, a smug expression, and a "you had it coming" attitude.

Our Lord gives second, third, and seventy-times-seven chances. He's the author of grace and redemption. He longs to heal and restore us. He is the loving Father who runs toward the prodigal child to welcome her home.

We simply live in a sin-stained world, and that means things don't work like they originally did. So husbands and wives aren't always on the same page about sexual desire.

We also have free will, meaning we can choose godly sexual intimacy in our marriage or choose less than that. Moreover, we have wounds from our past that impact how we address our current situation.

Until Jesus returns and reestablishes his full kingdom, we're subject to hardship and struggle no matter what we do. But we can seek out his superior ways and invite as much of his kingdom as we can into our marriage and bedroom.

Can I Leave a Sexless Marriage?

A sexless marriage is defined as having sex ten or fewer times a year. Sadly, some higher desire wives haven't had sex in months or even years. When someone shares a story like this, her emotional pain is palpable. I ache to sit with this wife, hold her in my arms, and say, "Yes, you deserve more."

But is a husband's refusal to engage sexually grounds for divorce?

Good Christians will disagree on this one. Most believe sexual unfaithfulness is a reason for divorce. But then the question becomes "What constitutes sexual unfaithfulness?" Is it just acting out sexually with another, or does it include failing one's marital duty to engage in physical intimacy?

Whatever I and others might think about the validity of divorce, I've never told someone to get one. For one thing, I don't have the whole story. It could be that a husband has good reasons to say no right now and he also wants something better but doesn't know where to begin. In any case, if someone wants to leave or to stay, my few words aren't likely to affect their decision.

But those aren't the only reasons. I'm also a believer in hope, redemption, and restoration; indeed, I'm the product of those things. When my marriage was terrible—and it really was a few years into our journey—things looked hopeless. But we found our way back and recently celebrated thirty-two years of marriage, most of which have been really good.

I cannot say whether you should leave or not, but I would say that you should give your marriage 100% before considering alternatives. Seek the counsel of trusted mentors, your pastor, a licensed counselor, and of course God in prayer. Give your valid feelings room for expression and the grieving process they deserve, but don't make final decisions based solely on hurt. Look at the overall picture of what marriage is and should be. Take the time and space needed to make a decision that you'll feel good about not just today but ten years from now and beyond.

All that said, *if you are in an abusive or emotionally destructive marriage, please get immediate help.* Keep yourself, and your children, safe. It's not God's will for us to tolerate oppression, no matter where it comes from! So if your husband is abusive, set boundaries and pursue healing for yourself.

Will It Ever Get Better?

While I wish I could turn to the last page of your story, read a happy ending, and then share the good news, I don't know how your story ends. God can take care of you, but beyond that I can't say how the sexual intimacy in your marriage will turn out. What I can say is that I've heard many success stories.

Couples who struggled with a desire gap for months or years or experienced conflict around sex contact me to say that they've found fresh, exciting intimacy. The change is rarely immediate but rather the culmination of at least one spouse's intentionality, ongoing kindness, and respect; the Spirit working in both husband and wife; and practical steps the couple has taken to make improvements.

My favorite emails come from elderly couples who now have the time and focus to savor one another's bodies and the pleasure and intimacy they bring. Many of them share stories of how things weren't always that good, but they're glad they held on and get regular glimpses of the intimacy God longs to have with us.

You don't need to wait until senior status to see positive changes! Great transformation is possible. In the next chapter, I'll share specific stories of success.

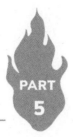

HOPE FOR
A HIGHER
DESIRE WIFE

I want higher desire wives to feel you're not alone but also empowered to improve the sexual intimacy in your marriage.

Now I want to leave you with even more hope. Hope built not on hollow platitudes or deceptive guarantees but on honest stories of success and your value in your own marriage story.

40. Stories of Success

Hopefully, you didn't turn here immediately, looking for guarantees. As much as I'd like to provide them, I can't give you what God himself won't. Jesus said, "Here on earth you will have many trials and sorrows" (John 16:33 NLT). That's a promise—this life isn't heaven, and we shouldn't expect it to be.

But Jesus also said, "I have come that they may have life, and have it to the full" (John 10:10), and "Come to me, all you who are weary and burdened, and I will give you rest" (Matt. 11:28). And in the John 16 verse cited above, he also reassured us, "Take heart, because I have overcome the world."

Success might involve a breakthrough in your marriage, in which sex becomes a priority for your husband and you both enjoy fantastic physical intimacy! But it might involve learning how to cope with the trials and sorrows of an imperfect world, finding rest in God, and taking heart because Christ's work is finished and your future is certain. Whatever intimacy you might experience here, it will pale in comparison to eternity in God's presence.

That doesn't make your hardship less. But we need to define success according to God's parameters, not our own.

Progress, Not Perfection

If I'd written a book titled *10 Surefire Ways to Get Your Husband to Pursue Sex*, I might sell more copies than this book. But I'd also be lying to you—something I refuse to do. I want to give realistic but achievable expectations. Your problems will not be resolved tomorrow, but growth is more than possible! It's been done by many couples before you, and it could be your story as well.

Rather than aiming at perfection, set your sights on progress.

For instance, while Naomi and her husband are still working their way through some issues, he's on a path of recovery from porn use and they've figured out how to engage better:

> We've grown as people. For example, my husband's been better at saying, "Hey, I want something tonight" or "It's not a good night for it. Can we do tomorrow or the day after?" Or I might say, "Hey, I'm interested tonight. What's something I could do to help you relieve some stress or be more interested?"
>
> Some of it for my husband was just taking the pressure off— maybe more being available than being all over him, learning to give him a couple days in between, and reworking my expectations. Like, *Okay, what I'm expecting might be unrealistic right now.*

Not perfect, but definitely progress.

My own marriage sucked twenty years ago. Like Hoover-vacuum-on-high sucked. I doubted we'd make it. Yet we're now past thirty years of marriage. Is it perfect? Nope. But is it good? Yes. By the grace of God, my marriage is solid and satisfying. It's more than enough.

Can I Get a Witness?

One of the joys of my ministry is hearing from those who've improved their sexual intimacy and thus their whole marriage. Consider a few more stories that may inspire you.

Babette. The turnaround in Babette's marriage came about fifteen years in, when her husband was working two jobs to clear family debt and she was aching for connection. She recounted to me, "It was kind of a come-to-Jesus moment that he realized what he was doing to me. It's like he finally woke up after all these years and stepped up a whole lot more."

That "aha" moment didn't resolve everything. They also embraced a sex schedule recommended on the *ONE Extraordinary Marriage* podcast. Hosts Tony and Alisa DiLorenzo describe their "intimacy lifestyle" as having windows of time (usually a few days) during which one spouse is expected to initiate, with other days of the week falling to the other spouse to initiate within that time frame.[1] Here's how Babette explained it:

> He can initiate on three days, and I can initiate on three days, and then we have one night where it's just a possibility. . . . So, it's still a surprise, but we know whose turn it is to initiate.
>
> It helps me because I was typically higher drive, so I knew I was going to get some, and he knew what the expectations were—that we needed to have it at least twice a week and sometimes three times a week.

Introducing structure to prioritize sexual intimacy and to set reasonable expectations helped this couple close their sexual desire gap.

Danita. Danita once initiated 80% of the time, but now she and her husband initiate equally. Part of her strategy has been to choose opportunities more likely to lead to success. "Before I was swinging at just about every pitch, versus now I'm kind of picking a little bit better."

Danita also recognized that her husband isn't that visual, but there are ways to appeal to his sexy side.

> The playful banter, like double entendres and stuff like that—that kind of tends to get him going a bit more. Kind of like the little stolen moments. Like when we're getting supper together for the kids and I grab his butt or stuff like that—what I would call still quite PG-13 type stuff, but around the house.

Learning her husband's makeup helped them negotiate sexual intimacy that's satisfying for them both.

Gail. Gail's sexual interest increased later in life, at the same time her husband's interest was lessening. But while her mind was eager-beaver, some autoimmune issues had made her genitals sleepy-sloth. That is, she'd lost sensation down there, especially with her clitoris. To address this factor, she began taking testosterone pellets. "I thought that was a miracle cure. The sensations were there for the first time in, I don't know, ten years or more."

But while she appreciated the reawakening, it made the sex drive gap with her husband wider. How did they close the gap? "I finally had to go to him in tears and just say, 'I need you to want me. I'm dying over here with all of these hormones.'"

She convinced him to check with his healthcare provider, and he got on T pellets as well. When I asked if they were matched now, her response was a massive grin.

Tara. I left Tara's story for last, perhaps because she and her husband had the most to overcome. Joe's childhood abuse was extreme and persistent, and its effect on their marriage was significant. The journey was difficult, including many tearful nights and learning what they each needed to move forward.

He was not ready in the early years to completely unearth to me the details. And then about seven years in is when he had, not a mental breakdown, but a coming apart at the seams where he began to truly deal with his childhood trauma. And that's when he was able for the first time to just sob into my arms and say, "I don't know why they did that to me. I don't know why they did that to me. . . . This hurts so bad. Why does this still hurt so much?"

It was the huge turning point of our marriage because then I was able to develop that empathy for him. And then suddenly me being hurt that he's pushing me away—I understood why.

So after that major breakthrough, we began to heal over the next five to ten years. And then every conversation we had or every fight we had, we were able to dig into a little deeper part of his story, and he was able to share more. We worked together to find solutions. He felt safer to begin to say more difficult things. . . . And sometimes he would tell me something, and all he needed to hear was, "Honey, that wasn't your fault."

That was just a turning point where we went the opposite direction, turning toward each other instead of away. It didn't all change right away. It was, *Okay, that was good*, and then, *That was better*. Then another year later, we'd get this other thing figured out. So we saw a turnaround, and he began to want to work with me, and he could identify his triggers more quickly. We had hope.

After ten-plus years of working on their sex life, Tara says it became "consistently good." They're now in their third decade of marriage and host the *Behind the Smiles* marriage podcast. Tara still identifies as the higher desire spouse, but the gap is small. She concluded by saying, "Sometimes I'm like, *We are having the time of our lives*. It took us twenty years to get there. But . . ."

Tara leaves off and just smiles. Well worth it.

What HDWs Want You to Know

One question I asked most HDWs I interviewed was, "What would you like other higher desire wives to know?" Their responses were so insightful, I simply want to share a few:

- "That you're not alone."
- "It's not your fault."
- "You're normal."
- "Speak up."
- "When you're feeling frustrated, go to God first. Start with prayer."
- "You don't have to stay stuck. God can redeem things."
- "You're beautiful. Who you are inside, your desires, your feelings are exactly who you're supposed to be and are

God-given. And even though you're in a difficult situation that can be heart-wrenching, just know that you're loved and you're beautiful and you're okay."

While I agree with all of those, what I most want you to take away from this book is in the final chapter. Let's turn the page.

41. The Value of a Wife

Elkanah was an Ephraimite married first to Hannah and then to Peninnah. Now, I already dislike something about this guy, because he took two wives when one should have been puh-lenty. But I don't know the whole story. Maybe he was obligated by his family to take that second wife, or she needed the protection of a husband, or without an heir from his first wife he worried his whole household was at risk of being overtaken. Whenever I read stories like this one, I try to imagine being in their culture, not mine. With that in mind, let's read about Elkanah. First Samuel 1:4–8 explains,

> When the day came that Elkanah sacrificed, he would give portions to his wife Peninnah and to all her sons and daughters; but to Hannah he would give a double portion, because he loved Hannah, but the LORD had closed her womb. Her rival, moreover, would provoke her bitterly to irritate her, because the LORD had closed her womb. And it happened year after year, as often as she went up to the house of the LORD, that she would provoke her; so she wept and would not eat. Then Elkanah her husband would say to her, "Hannah, why do you weep, and why do you not eat, and why is your heart sad? Am I not better to you than ten sons?" (NASB)

In that culture, Peninnah, with all her children, should have been the prize wife, but Elkanah "loved Hannah" and gave her a double portion. He also reassured her that he'd care for her no matter what—"better . . . than ten sons."

Yet Hannah did not have what she most wanted, a child. Her longing for a child was not only understandable but good. "Children are a heritage from the LORD, offspring a reward from him" (Ps. 127:3). You probably know the rest of the story: how she prayed to God in the temple, how Eli the priest blessed her, and how she conceived Samuel and dedicated him to the Lord. But Hannah didn't need any of that to have value in the eyes of her husband or the heart of God. Elkanah knew that "charm is deceptive, and beauty is fleeting; but a woman who fears the LORD"— like Hannah—"is to be praised" (Prov. 31:30).

You, higher desire wife, don't have something you want, and your longing for it is good. I've written this book with the hope that your story turns out like Hannah's: with the reassurance of a husband who loves you, the fulfillment of that longing, and dedication of that blessing to the Lord.

But even before any progress is made, you are valuable. With or without a rockin' sex life, you're a sensual being, made in God's image, and, I hope and pray, a woman who fears the Lord.

Is He Your Elkanah?

Your husband probably doesn't feel to you like an Elkanah right now. (Although be glad he didn't take that second wife. You've got enough on your plate already, right?) You wish he'd reassure you of his love. You long for a double portion of his goodness to at least try to make up for the lack of sexual satisfaction in your marriage. You also know that nothing can satisfy this deep desire for intimacy like a healthy and holy sex life with him. As Proverbs 13:12 says, "Hope deferred makes the heart sick, but a longing fulfilled is a tree of life."

But what if he is Elkanah? What if he's also frustrated by the situation? Unsure how to sate that longing? Frustrated by his lack of drive? Feeling that he cannot—for whatever reason—give you what you desire right now? What if he loves you but doesn't feel he can make things right?

That's where a lot of lower desire husbands are. Yes, some don't care all that much, in which case you have not just a sex problem but also a marriage problem. But many husbands have deferred hope and sick hearts as well.

You Can Be a Hero

Even after her fervent prayer and Eli's blessings, Hannah's longing was not immediately fulfilled. According to 1 Samuel 1:20, "In the course of time Hannah became pregnant and gave birth to a son." It did not happen right away, but *in the course of time.*

We HDWs are understandably impatient, but Hannah did not give up. Nor should we.

In fact, Elkanah is by no means the only hero in this story. Hannah champions goodness for her family and faithfulness in God.

Perhaps you, too, are the hero in your story, the one who nudges your marriage bit by bit to a healthier place that includes sexual intimacy as God intended. In the course of time.

You have value as a wife in many other ways, but you add value in the sex department as well if you're the catalyst for positive change. Excellent wife, take what you've learned in this book, apply it with gentleness and love, and build better marital intimacy.

> An excellent wife, who can find her?
> For her worth is far above jewels. (Prov. 31:10 NASB)

Acknowledgments

Penning a book isn't an easy endeavor, but this page always strikes me as the most difficult to write. It's impossible to thank everyone who brought me to this place, and simply hitting the highlights makes me worry that I've forgotten someone important. Yet here I go!

A big thank-you to the higher desire wives who allowed me to interview them and to include their stories in this book. Your authenticity and wisdom brought so much to this project. Also, thanks to those women who read my first draft and offered valuable suggestions.

Cheers to Patnacia Goodman, who acquired this project for Baker Books, and to the other staff at Baker who've tended my book with such dedication—Jessica, Rachel, Shari, Sarah, Brianna, Eileen, and [insert your name and my apology here]. And thanks to my lovely agent, Karen Neumair, who believed that I was the one to write this book and who continues to pursue books that empower women.

Thanks to colleagues who added to my knowledge and encouraged me on this project, especially Juli Slattery, whose response when I pitched this book was "Yes, you should write it. That's so needed." Her reassurance came back to me many times over and kept me going. (That's also a reminder, folks, that you never know when the small praise you give yields a big impact for the one who hears it.)

Speaking of colleagues, many thanks to my *Sex Chat for Christian Wives* cohosts—Bonny Burns, Gaye Christmus, and Chris Taylor—who've supported me both professionally and personally for well over the seven years we've podcasted together.

And here's to all of you higher desire men who told me that higher desire wives were a myth or their husbands must be broken, because that just motivated me to get the truth out! You're wrong, I'm right, and frankly, that feels good. [grin] But as I remind myself (yet again) that humility is one of the best virtues, I should say that I'm mostly just glad that the conversation in Christian churches and circles is shifting so that everyone will come to appreciate the prevalence and normality of higher desire wives and lower desire husbands.

Finally, thanks to my husband and to God—not in that order. But without my husband's support, I couldn't have written any books, much less this passion project that took years to finish. Moreover, he always gave me a thumbs-up to talk about him being the lower desire spouse and never once believed it diminished his masculinity or his sexuality. Ultimately, though, our beautiful sexual intimacy is all due to God, who worked in our lives to bring us to this point.

Lord, thank you for everything. Please use my imperfect words to bring your truth to those who need it and, through your Holy Spirit, enable couples to pursue intimacy in the bedroom that strengthens marriages and honors you.

Notes

Chapter 1 How Many of Us Are There?

1. Shaunti Feldhahn, *The Good News about Marriage: Debunking Discouraging Myths about Marriage and Divorce* (Colorado Springs: Multnomah, 2014), 20.

2. Christopher Quinn-Nilas, "Midlife Sex Problems? New Research Says You're Not Alone," The Conversation, June 22, 2020, https://theconversation .com/midlife-sex-problems-new-research-says-youre-not-alone-101023.

3. Roy F. Baumeister, Kathleen R. Catanese, and Kathleen D. Vohs, "Is There a Gender Difference in Strength of Sex Drive? Theoretical Views, Conceptual Distinctions, and a Review of Relevant Evidence," *Personality and Social Psychology Review* 5, no. 3 (2001): 242–73, https://doi.org/10.1207/s15327957pspr0503_5.

4. Natalie O. Rosen, Kristen Bailey, and Amy Muise, "Degree and Direction of Sexual Desire Discrepancy Are Linked to Sexual and Relationship Satisfaction in Couples Transitioning to Parenthood," *Journal of Sex Research* 55, no. 2 (2018): 214–25, https://www.tandfonline.com/doi/full/10.1080/00224499 .2017.1321732.

5. Cynthia A. Graham et al., "What Factors Are Associated with Reporting Lacking Interest in Sex and How Do These Vary by Gender? Findings from the Third British National Survey of Sexual Attitudes and Lifestyles," *BMJ Open* 7, no. 9 (2017), https://doi.org/10.1136/bmjopen-2017-016942.

6. Chloe Tejada, "Women Want More Sex Than Their Partner Does, According to New Study," HuffPost, August 21, 2017, https://www.huffpost.com/archive /ca/entry/women-high-sex-drive-a_23155678.

7. Shaunti Feldhahn and Michael Sytsma, *Secrets of Sex and Marriage: 8 Surprises That Make All the Difference* (Minneapolis: Bethany House, 2023), 111.

8. Admittedly, this research focuses on the United States, the United Kingdom, and Canada. Well-sampled and reviewed studies from various countries and cultures would be helpful in determining not only how prevalent higher desire wives are but how societal factors play a role in our expectations and experiences.

9. Veera Korhonen, "Number of Married Couples in the United States from 1960 to 2022," Statista, July 5, 2024, https://www.statista.com/statistics/183663/number-of-married-couples-in-the-us/; "Census Bureau Releases Report on Same-Sex Couple Households," United States Census Bureau, February 24, 2021, https://www.census.gov/newsroom/press-releases/2021/same-sex-couple-households.html.

Chapter 4 Low Testosterone

1. E. Cirino, "All about Testosterone in Women," Healthline, June 10, 2019, https://www.healthline.com/health/womens-health/do-women-have-testosterone.

2. " Howard E. LeWine, ed., "Testosterone: What It Is and How It Affects Your Health," Harvard Health Publishing, June 22, 2023, https://www.health.harvard.edu/staying-healthy/testosterone--what-it-does-and-doesnt-do.

3. "Testosterone," Mount Sinai Health System, accessed March 24, 2022, https://www.mountsinai.org/health-library/tests/testosterone.

4. "Testosterone, Free, Direct," Labcorp, accessed March 24, 2022, https://www.labcorp.com/tests/144980/testosterone-free-direct.

5. Daniel Kelly, "Testosterone: Why Defining a 'Normal' Level Is Hard to Do," The Conversation, January 20, 2022, https://theconversation.com/testosterone-why-defining-a-normal-level-is-hard-to-do-113587.

6. Jayne Leonard, "What Are the Signs of High Testosterone in Males?," Medical News Today, MediLexicon International, February 9, 2023, https://www.medicalnewstoday.com/articles/signs-of-high-testosterone.

7. "Testosterone Therapy: Potential Benefits and Risks as You Age," Mayo Clinic, accessed January 19, 2024, https://www.mayoclinic.org/healthy-lifestyle/sexual-health/in-depth/testosterone-therapy/art-20045728.

8. Alvin M. Matsumoto, ed., "The Truth about Testosterone Treatments," Endocrine Society, accessed March 29, 2022, https://www.endocrine.org/-/media/endocrine/files/patient-engagement/patient-guides/patient_guide_the_truth_about_testosterone_treatments.pdf.

Chapter 5 His Weight

1. Jamin Brahmbhatt, quoted in Macaela Mackenzie, "6 Ways Your Diet Is Destroying Your Sex Life," Men's Health, February 8, 2018, https://www.menshealth.com/health/a19547196/how-diet-affects-sex-life/.

2. Robert Krysiak, Witold Szkróbka, and Bogusław Okopień, "Sexual Functioning and Depressive Symptoms in Men with Various Types of Prediabetes: A Pilot Study," *International Journal of Impotence Research* 30 (2018): 327–34, https://doi.org/10.1038/s41443-018-0050-6.

3. *The Late Late Show*, "Michael Bublé Carpool Karaoke," YouTube video, October 26, 2018, https://www.youtube.com/watch?v=Kg7UWnNF_rA.

Chapter 6 His Diet

1. Lisa M. Caronia et al., "Abrupt Decrease in Serum Testosterone Levels After an Oral Glucose Load in Men: Implications for Screening for Hypogonadism," *Clinical Endocrinology* 78, no. 2 (February 2013): 291–96, https://doi.org/10.1111/j.1365-2265.2012.04486.x; Thiago Gagliano-Jucá et al., "Oral Glucose Load and

Mixed Meal Feeding Lowers Testosterone Levels in Healthy Eugonadal Men,"
Endocrine 63 (2019): 149–56, https://doi.org/10.1007/s12020-018-1741-y.

Chapter 7 Alcohol and Drugs

1. "Othello," Folger Shakespeare Library, accessed August 19, 2024, https://www.folger.edu/explore/shakespeares-works/othello/.

2. Macaela Mackenzie, "6 Ways Your Diet Is Destroying Your Sex Life," Men's Health, February 8, 2018, https://www.menshealth.com/health/a19547196/how-diet-affects-sex-life/.

3. Tim Jewell, "Risk Factors of Having High or Low Estrogen Levels in Males," Healthline, March 16, 2023, https://www.healthline.com/health/estrogen-in-men#high-estrogen.

4. "The Basics: Defining How Much Alcohol Is Too Much," National Institute on Alcohol Abuse and Alcoholism, accessed May 10, 2023, https://www.niaaa.nih.gov/health-professionals-communities/core-resource-on-alcohol/basics-defining-how-much-alcohol-too-much.

5. "Is Marijuana Addictive?," National Institute on Drug Abuse, accessed June 28, 2024, https://nida.nih.gov/publications/research-reports/marijuana/marijuana-addictive.

6. Amanda Moser et al., "The Influence of Cannabis on Sexual Functioning and Satisfaction," *Journal of Cannabis Research* 5, no. 2 (2023), https://doi.org/10.1186/s42238-022-00169-2.

7. Ann Pietrangelo, "The Effects of Marijuana on Your Body," Healthline, April 27, 2021, https://www.healthline.com/health/effects-of-cannabis-on-body.

8. Dispensaries.com, "Is Marijuana Good for Sex, Bad for Sperm?," MySA, January 3, 2019, https://www.mysanantonio.com/news/article/Is-Marijuana-Good-for-Sex-Bad-for-Sperm-13506346.php.

9. "Drug Overdose Death Rates," National Institute on Drug Abuse, accessed June 28, 2024, https://nida.nih.gov/research-topics/trends-statistics/overdose-death-rates.

10. Jamie Eske, "What Are the Effects of Drug Misuse?," Medical News Today, February 14, 2023, https://www.medicalnewstoday.com/articles/effects-of-drug-abuse.

11. D. S. Ghadigaonkar and P. Murthy, "Sexual Dysfunction in Persons with Substance Use Disorders," *Journal of Psychosexual Health* 1, no. 2 (2019): 117–21, https://doi.org/10.1177/2631831819849365.

12. "Al-Anon's Three Cs—I Didn't Cause It, I Can't Control It, and I Can't Cure It—Removed the Blame . . ." Al-Anon Family Groups, accessed June 28, 2024, https://al-anon.org/blog/al-anons-three-cs/.

13. Dr. Gregory Jantz, "Married to an Addict: How to Help Your Loved One," Focus on the Family, March 14, 2022, https://www.focusonthefamily.com/marriage/married-to-an-addict-how-to-help-your-loved-one/.

Chapter 8 His Sleep

1. Monica Levy Andersen and Sergio Tufik, "The Effects of Testosterone on Sleep and Sleep-Disordered Breathing in Men: Its Bidirectional Interaction with Erectile Function," *Sleep Medicine Reviews* 12, no. 5 (October 2008): 365–79, https://doi.org/10.1016/j.smrv.2007.12.003.

2. Lee Smith et al., "Sleep Quality, Duration, and Associated Sexual Function at Older Age: Findings from the English Longitudinal Study of Ageing," *Journal of Sexual Medicine* 16, no. 3 (March 2019): 427–33, https://doi.org/10.1016/j.jsxm.2019.01.005.

3. "Moderation in All Things," Oxford Reference, accessed August 19, 2024, https://www.oxfordreference.com/display/10.1093/oi/authority.20110810105420435.

4. Zoe Miller, "Sleep and Testosterone Levels: What's the Connection?," TRTed, accessed March 23, 2024, https://www.trted.org/articles/sleep-and-testosterone-levels-whats-the-connection; Taylor P. Kohn et al., "The Effect of Sleep on Men's Health," *Translational Andrology and Urology* 9, no. 2 (March 5, 2020), https://doi.org/10.21037/tau.2019.11.07.

5. R. Leproult and Eve Van Cauter, "Effect of 1 Week of Sleep Restriction on Testosterone Levels in Young Healthy Men," *JAMA* 305, no. 21 (June 1, 2011): 2173–74, https://jamanetwork.com/journals/jama/fullarticle/1029127.

6. Michael Monostra, "Sleep Duration May Affect Testosterone Levels for Men and Women Differently by Age," Healio, August 8, 2023, https://www.healio.com/news/endocrinology/20230807/sleep-duration-may-affect-testosterone-levels-for-men-and-women-differently-by-age.

7. Warren Fields, "Lack of Sleep Can Lower Men's Libido and Semen Levels," Men's Variety, June 28, 2019, https://mensvariety.com/sleep-lower-semen-levels/.

8. As someone with sleep apnea, I testify to feeling better rested after I got my continuous positive airway pressure (CPAP) machine. In case someone's reluctant to go that route, yes, it's awkward the first few nights, but after that . . . no big deal. And while I might look weird to my husband with tubes around my face, he considers me even more appealing when I'm not snoring like a lumberjack sawing logs.

9. "Sleep Disorders," Mayo Clinic, accessed August 10, 2019, https://www.mayoclinic.org/diseases-conditions/sleep-disorders/symptoms-causes/syc-20354018.

10. Danielle Pacheco, "The Best Temperature for Sleep," Sleep Foundation, March 7, 2024, https://www.sleepfoundation.org/bedroom-environment/best-temperature-for-sleep.

Chapter 9 Aging

1. "Testosterone, Aging, and the Mind," Harvard Medical School, January 1, 2008, https://www.health.harvard.edu/newsletter_article/testosterone_aging_and_the_mind.

2. "Benign Prostatic Hyperplasia," Mount Sinai Health System, accessed June 8, 2023, https://www.mountsinai.org/health-library/report/benign-prostatic-hyperplasia.

3. "Enlarged Prostate: Medlineplus Medical Encyclopedia," MedlinePlus, accessed July 1, 2023, https://medlineplus.gov/ency/article/000381.htm.

4. "Dry Orgasm," Mayo Clinic, accessed November 30, 2022, https://www.mayoclinic.org/symptoms/dry-orgasm/basics/definition/sym-20050906.

5. I recommend MarriedDance.com, which is owned by a Christian husband-wife team and provides marriage-focused instructions for their products.

6. Robert Browning, "Rabbi Ben Ezra," Poetry Foundation, accessed September 12, 2023, https://www.poetryfoundation.org/poems/43775/rabbi-ben-ezra.

Chapter 11 Ongoing Pain

1. Michael Silberman et al., "Priapism," StatPearls, May 30, 2023, https://www.ncbi.nlm.nih.gov/books/NBK459178/.

2. "Peyronie Disease," Mayo Clinic, accessed December 1, 2023, https://www.mayoclinic.org/diseases-conditions/peyronies-disease/symptoms-causes/syc-20353468.

3. Jerry Kennard, "Infections and Foreskin Problems Put Men at Risk during Sex," Verywell Health, January 5, 2024, https://www.verywellhealth.com/pain-during-intercourse-2329078.

Personal History

1. "The Tempest," Folger Shakespeare Library, accessed July 1, 2024, https://www.folger.edu/explore/shakespeares-works/the-tempest/read/.

Chapter 12 Poor Modeling

1. "We Don't Talk about Bruno" is a popular song from the Disney movie *Encanto*, in which various characters sing about not bringing up a family member they haven't seen in a while because doing so might bring bad results. (See "We Don't Talk about Bruno," track 4 on *Encanto [Original Motion Picture Soundtrack]*, Disney, 2021.)

Chapter 13 Purity Messaging

1. Joe Carter, "The FAQs: What You Should Know about Purity Culture," The Gospel Coalition, July 24, 2019, https://www.thegospelcoalition.org/article/faqs-know-purity-culture/.

2. Gary Smalley and Ted Cunningham, *The Language of Sex: Experiencing the Beauty of Sexual Intimacy* (Ventura, CA: Regal, 2008), 130.

3. Cambridge Dictionary, s.v. "repression," accessed March 10, 2022, https://dictionary.cambridge.org/us/dictionary/english/repression#google_vignette (emphasis added).

Chapter 14 Prior Relationships

1. "Your fill" is also translated as "drunk" or "intoxicated." The husband and wife in Song of Songs are encouraged to go overboard with caresses, intimacy, and expressions of love. What a generous Father we have!

Chapter 15 Childhood Abuse

1. "11 Facts about Child Abuse," DoSomething.org, accessed November 7, 2023, https://www.dosomething.org/us/facts/11-facts-about-child-abuse.
2. Bessel van der Kolk, *The Body Keeps the Score: Brain, Mind, and Body in the Healing of Trauma* (New York: Penguin Books, 2015), 2.
3. Van der Kolk, *The Body Keeps the Score*, 3.
4. Van der Kolk, *The Body Keeps the Score*, 86.

Chapter 16 Body Image

1. This saying is often misattributed to Theodore Roosevelt, when the earliest exact match comes from a 2004 book written by Curt Cloninger, who simply included it as "Somebody once said that comparison is the thief of joy." (Quote Investigator, "Comparison Is the Thief of Joy," February 6, 2021, https://quote investigator.com/2021/02/06/thief-of-joy/.)
2. J. Lever, D. A. Frederick, and L. A. Peplau, "Does Size Matter? Men's and Women's Views on Penis Size across the Lifespan," *Psychology of Men & Masculinity*, https://psycnet.apa.org/doiLanding?doi=10.1037%2F1524-9220.7.3.129. A survey sample collected through the internet, especially in 2006, may be a bit skewed, but the results are consistent with other studies' findings.
3. "What Size Is the Average Penis?," Medical News Today, accessed June 12, 2023, https://www.medicalnewstoday.com/articles/271647#when-is-penis-size -too-small.
4. AFP and Amanda Macias, "Scientists Measured 15,000 Penises and Determined the Average Size," Business Insider, March 3, 2015, https://www.business insider.com/afp-penis-size-researchers-provide-the-long-and-short-of-it-2015-3.
5. Lever, Frederick, and Peplau, "Does Size Matter?"
6. Nicole Prause et al., "Women's Preferences for Penis Size: A New Research Method Using Selection among 3D Models," PLOS ONE, September 2, 2015, https://journals.plos.org/plosone/article?id=10.1371%2Fjournal.pone.0133079.
7. Lever, Frederick, and Peplau, "Does Size Matter?"

Chapter 17 Fatherhood Fears

1. I highly recommend this resource: Sarah E. Hill, *This Is Your Brain on Birth Control: The Surprising Science of Women, Hormones, and the Law of Unintended Consequences* (New York: Avery, 2019).
2. S. K. Nelson et al., "In Defense of Parenthood: Children Are Associated with More Joy Than Misery," *Psychological Science* 24, no. 1 (November 30, 2012): 3–10, https://doi.org/10.1177/0956797612447798; Roy F. Baumeister et al., "Some Key Differences between a Happy Life and a Meaningful Life," *Journal of Positive Psychology* 8, no. 6 (August 20, 2013): 505–16, https://doi.org/10.1080/17439760.2013.830764.

Chapter 18 Depression and Anxiety

1. "Patient Health Questionnaire," Patient, accessed July 15, 2024, https://patient.info/doctor/patient-health-questionnaire-phq-9.

2. Mayo Clinic Staff, "Male Depression: Understanding the Issues," Mayo Clinic, accessed July 15, 2024, https://www.mayoclinic.org/diseases-conditions/depression/in-depth/male-depression/art-20046216.

3. "Impact of the DSM-IV to DSM-5 Changes on the National Survey on Drug Use and Health," National Library of Medicine, June 2016, https://www.ncbi.nlm.nih.gov/books/NBK519704/table/ch3.t15/.

4. "How Anxiety Impacts Men versus Women," UNC School of Medicine, accessed July 15, 2024, https://www.med.unc.edu/menshealth/how-anxiety-impacts-men-versus-women/.

Chapter 19 Stress

1. Hedy Marks and Lori M. King, "Stress Symptoms," WebMD, June 19, 2024, https://www.webmd.com/balance/stress-management/stress-symptoms-effects_of-stress-on-the-body.

2. Marks and King, "Stress Symptoms."

3. Peter Morales-Brown, "Does Sex Provide Health Benefits?," Medical News Today, November 22, 2023, https://www.medicalnewstoday.com/articles/316954.

4. "Understanding the Stress Response: Chronic Activation of This Survival Mechanism Impairs Health," Harvard Health, April 3, 2024, https://www.health.harvard.edu/staying-healthy/understanding-the-stress-response.

5. Daniel A. Cox, "Men's Social Circles Are Shrinking," Survey Center on American Life, June 29, 2021, https://www.americansurveycenter.org/why-mens-social-circles-are-shrinking/.

Chapter 20 Psychiatric Disorders

1. Michael McDonough, "5 Common Misconceptions about Schizophrenia," Encyclopaedia Britannica, accessed March 26, 2024, https://www.britannica.com/list/5-common-misconceptions-about-schizophrenia.

2. "Understanding Psychosis," National Institute of Mental Health, accessed March 26, 2024, https://www.nimh.nih.gov/health/publications/understanding-psychosis#.

3. Sebastián Vargas-Cáceres et al., "The Impact of Psychosis on Sexual Functioning: A Systematic Review," *Journal of Sexual Medicine* 18, no. 3 (March 2021): 457–66, https://doi.org/10.1016/j.jsxm.2020.12.007.

4. L. J. Thana et al., "Barriers to the Management of Sexual Dysfunction among People with Psychosis: Analysis of Qualitative Data from the REMEDY Trial," *BMC Psychiatry* 22, no. 545 (2022), https://doi.org/10.1186/s12888-022-04193-7.

5. "Post-Traumatic Stress Disorder (PTSD)," Mayo Clinic, accessed December 13, 2022, https://www.mayoclinic.org/diseases-conditions/post-traumatic-stress-disorder/symptoms-causes/syc-20355967.

6. Elizabeth R. Bird et al., "Relationship between Posttraumatic Stress Disorder and Sexual Difficulties: A Systematic Review of Veterans and Military Personnel," *Journal of Sexual Medicine* 18, no. 8 (August 2021): 1398–426, https://doi.org/10.1016/j.jsxm.2021.05.011.

7. "Fact Sheet: Sexual Abuse of Boys," Prevent Child Abuse America, accessed November 2, 2023, https://preventchildabuse.org/images/docs/sexualabuseofboys.pdf.

8. Diana Rodriguez, "Hypersexuality and Bipolar Disorder: When Impulsive Sexual Behavior Is Part of a Manic Episode," EverydayHealth.com, August 21, 2023, https://www.everydayhealth.com/bipolar-disorder/bipolar-disorder-and-sex .aspx; Jon Johnson, "What to Know about Bipolar Disorder and Sex," Medical News Today, March 1, 2019, https://www.medicalnewstoday.com/articles/324595.

Chapter 21 Sexual Orientation and Identity

1. I'm not going to address the scientific, sociological, philosophical, or moral views of sexual orientation in this chapter. While I have biblically based opinions, it's not my mission here to dive into that question, and such a discussion would be a rabbit trail from the subject at hand. While you may have strong opinions about homosexuality, I encourage you to focus with me on the consequences a husband's view of his sexuality has on a marriage, which is the focus of this text.

2. Justin McCarthy, "Americans Still Greatly Overestimate U.S. Gay Population," Gallup, June 27, 2019, https://news.gallup.com/poll/259571/americans -greatly-overestimate-gay-population.aspx.

3. Texas has 9% of the US general population. (Taylor Orth, "From Millionaires to Muslims, Small Subgroups of the Population Seem Much Larger to Many Americans," YouGov, March 15, 2022, https://today.yougov.com/topics/politics/ar ticles-reports/2022/03/15/americans-misestimate-small-subgroups-population.)

4. McCarthy, "Americans Still Greatly Overestimate U.S. Gay Population."

5. *Seinfeld*, season 4, episode 17, "The Outing," directed by Tom Cherones, aired February 11, 1993, on NBC.

Chapter 22 Extramarital Sex

1. "Signs They're Having an Affair," WebMD, December 4, 2022, https:// www.webmd.com/sex-relationships/signs-theyre-having-affair; Korin Miller and Shannen Zitz, "19 Warning Signs Your Partner Is Cheating on You, According to Therapists," Prevention, October 16, 2023, https://www.prevention.com/sex /relationships/g26267590/signs-of-cheating-partner/.

Chapter 23 Pornography

1. Proven Men Ministries Ltd., "2014 Survey: How Many Christians Do You Think Watch Porn?" PR Newswire, August 14, 2014, https://www.prnewswire .com/news-releases/2014-survey-how-many-christians-do-you-think-watch-porn -271236741.html.

2. "The Porn Phenomenon," Barna, accessed June 9, 2023, https://www.barna .com/the-porn-phenomenon/.

3. Robert Weiss, "Understanding Porn-Induced Erectile Dysfunction (PIED)," HuffPost, August 24, 2017, https://www.huffpost.com/entry/understanding-porn induced_b_11668932.

4. Bonny Logsdon Burns, personal interview with author, October 23, 2023.

5. "New Report Reveals Truths about How Teens Engage with Pornography," Common Sense Media, January 10, 2023, https://www.commonsensemedia

.org/press-releases/new-report-reveals-truths-about-how-teens-engage-with
-pornography.

6. "The Porn Phenomenon."

7. NM, "Childhood Emotional Wounds: How They Affect Us as Adults," SouthEnd Psychiatry, February 9, 2022, https://southendpsych.com/childhood -emotional-wounds-how-they-affect-us-as-adults/.

8. Burns, personal interview.

9. Burns, personal interview.

10. Burns, personal interview.

Chapter 24 Sexual Acting Out

1. J. Parker, "Q&A with J: 'What Should We Call Persistent Porn Use?'" *Hot, Holy & Humorous*, August 19, 2017, https://hotholyhumorous.com/2017/03/09 /qa-with-j-what-should-we-call-persistent-porn-use/.

2. Maria Trimarchi and Ann Meeker-O'Connell, "How Nicotine Works," How Stuff Works, accessed August 15, 2023, https://science.howstuffworks.com/nicotine3 .htm.

3. "6C72 Compulsive Sexual Behaviour Disorder," ICD-11 for Mortality and Morbidity Statistics, January 2024, https://icd.who.int/browse/2024-01/mms/en #1630268048.

4. Sophie Scott, "Understanding Why We Do What We Do," ABC News, March 6, 2017, https://www.abc.net.au/news/health/2017-03-06/understanding -why-we-do-what-we-do/8322024; Society for Personality and Social Psychology, "How We Form Habits, Change Existing Ones," ScienceDaily, accessed March 28, 2024, https://www.sciencedaily.com/releases/2014/08/140808111931.htm.

5. Jay Stringer, *Unwanted: How Sexual Brokenness Reveals Our Way to Healing* (Colorado Springs: NavPress, 2018), xxi.

Chapter 25 Lack of Attraction

1. Kaz Cooke, *Real Gorgeous: The Truth about Body and Beauty* (New York: W. W. Norton, 1996), 140.

Chapter 27 And Baby Makes Three

1. Charles Dickens, *The Life and Adventures of Martin Chuzzlewit* (1853; Project Gutenberg, 2006), chap. 18, https://www.gutenberg.org/ebooks/968.

Chapter 28 His Passivity

1. Dictionary.com, s.v. "passive," accessed April 8, 2024, https://www.diction ary.com/browse/passive.

2. "Vitamin D," Harvard T.H. Chan School of Public Health, March 2023, https://www.hsph.harvard.edu/nutritionsource/vitamin-d/.

Chapter 29 Screen Time

1. Eileen Brown, "Americans Spend Far More Time on Their Smartphones Than They Think," ZDNET, April 28, 2019, https://www.zdnet.com/article /americans-spend-far-more-time-on-their-smartphones-than-they-think/.

2. Josh Howarth, "Alarming Average Screen Time Statistics (2024)," Exploding Topics, December 4, 2023, https://explodingtopics.com/blog/screen-time-stats.

3. Howarth, "Alarming Average Screen Time Statistics (2024)."

4. AnnaMarie Houlis, "This Is the Amount of Alone Time You Need to Save Your Relationship, According to Experts," Fairygodboss, accessed May 1, 2023, https://renderer.fairygodboss.com/career-topics/how-much-time-you-should-spend-with-your-partner-each-week-for-a-happy-relationship.

5. Sarah M. Flood and Katie R. Genadek, "Time for Each Other: Work and Family Constraints Among Couples," *Journal of Marriage and Family* 78, vol. 1 (February 2016): 142–64, https://doi.org/10.1111/jomf.12255.

6. Flood and Genadek, "Time for Each Other."

7. Andrea Sansone et al., "Relationship between Use of Videogames and Sexual Health in Adult Males," *Journal of Sexual Medicine* 14, no. 7 (July 2017): 898–903, https://doi.org/10.1016/j.jsxm.2017.05.001.

8. Paige Brettingen, "How Video Games Are Making You Bad in Bed," LEAFtv, December 13, 2021, https://www.leaf.tv/13400159/how-video-games-are-making-you-bad-in-bed/.

Chapter 31 Just Mismatched

1. Corey Allan, "Sexual Desire Differences: What If There's Nothing Going Wrong?," *Hot, Holy & Humorous*, December 10, 2012, https://hotholyhumorous.com/2012/12/10/sexual-desire-differences-what-if-theres-nothing-going-wrong/.

Chapter 32 What's Healthy and Holy?

1. Nancy Shute, "Is Sex Once a Week Enough for a Happy Relationship?," NPR, November 18, 2015, https://www.npr.org/sections/health-shots/2015/11/18/456482701/is-sex-once-a-week-enough-for-a-happy-relationship; Jay Cardiello, "What Is the Normal Sex Frequency by Age?" Verywell Health, August 22, 2024, https://www.verywellhealth.com/how-often-do-couples-really-have-sex-2329045; Tracey Cox, "How Many Times a Week Should You REALLY Be Having Sex? Tracey Cox Reveals the Perfect Number for a Happy Relationship," Daily Mail, April 13, 2016, https://www.dailymail.co.uk/femail/article-3536424/How-times-week-REALLY-having-sex.html.

Chapter 33 Higher Desire Wives in the Bible

1. "Kosher Sex," Judaism 101, accessed March 31, 2024, https://www.jewfaq.org/kosher_sex.

Chapter 34 Communicating About Sex

1. Stephen R. Covey, *The 7 Habits of Highly Effective People*, rev. ed. (New York: Free Press, 2004), 237.

2. Ellen Boeder, "Emotional Safety Is Necessary for Emotional Connection," The Gottman Institute, accessed March 5, 2024, https://www.gottman.com/blog/emotional-safety-is-necessary-for-emotional-connection/.

Chapter 35 Engaging Your Husband

1. Rosemary Basson, "The Female Sexual Response: A Different Model," *Journal of Sex & Marital Therapy* 26, vol. 1 (February 2, 2011): 51–65, https://doi.org/10.1080/009262300278641.

Chapter 36 Initiating Intimacy

1. CSU Fullerton HCOM, "Deborah Tannen: Gender-Specific Language Rituals," YouTube, December 27, 2013, https://www.youtube.com/watch?v=tUxnBZxsfoU&feature=youtu.be.
2. J. Parker, "He Doesn't Wanna, but I Do! Be the Brownie," *Hot, Holy & Humorous*, August 16, 2023, https://hotholyhumorous.com/2012/04/30/he-doesnt-wanna-but-i-do-be-the-brownie/.
3. Parker, "He Doesn't Wanna, but I Do!"

Chapter 37 Dealing with Rejection

1. J. Parker, "How the Sexually Rejected Spouse Feels," *Hot, Holy & Humorous*, July 2, 2020, https://hotholyhumorous.com/2019/10/15/how-rejected-spouse-feels/.

Chapter 38 Embracing Your Desire

1. "What Does It Mean to Stand in the Gap (Ezekiel 22:30)?," Got Questions, accessed July 22, 2024, https://www.gotquestions.org/stand-in-the-gap.html.

Chapter 39 FAQs for HDWs

1. Nancy Shute, "Is Sex Once a Week Enough for a Happy Relationship?," NPR, November 18, 2015, https://www.npr.org/sections/health-shots/2015/11/18/456482701/is-sex-once-a-week-enough-for-a-happy-relationship; Jay Cardiello, "What Is the Normal Sex Frequency by Age?" Verywell Health, August 22, 2024, https://www.verywellhealth.com/how-often-do-couples-really-have-sex-2329045; Tracey Cox, "How Many Times a Week Should You REALLY Be Having Sex? Tracey Cox Reveals the Perfect Number for a Happy Relationship," Daily Mail, April 13, 2016, https://www.dailymail.co.uk/femail/article-3536424/How-times-week-REALLY-having-sex.html.

Chapter 40 Stories of Success

1. Tony and Alisa DiLorenzo, "Scheduling Sex . . ." *ONE Extraordinary Marriage*, accessed January 29, 2021, https://oneextraordinarymarriage.com/scheduling-sex-a-quick-intimacy-lifestyle-overview/.

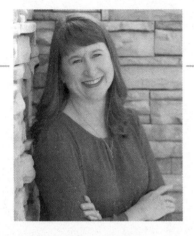

J. PARKER has been blogging at *Hot, Holy & Humorous* for nearly fifteen years and has written five books on sexual intimacy in marriage, including *Hot, Holy, and Humorous: Sex in Marriage by God's Design*. She holds a master's degree in counseling, but her personal testimony fueled her desire to write about God's design for sex in marriage. She fosters a Higher Desire Wives subscription community and cohosts *Sex Chat for Christian Wives*, a popular podcast about marriage and sexuality. She has two grown sons and one daughter-in-law and lives with her husband in the great state of Texas.

CONNECT WITH THE AUTHOR:

🌐 HotHolyHumorous.com   📷 @HotHolyHumorous

📘 @HotHolyAndHumorous   ✖ @HotHolyHumorous

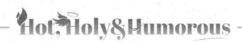

Hot, Holy & Humorous